W9-BYI-230

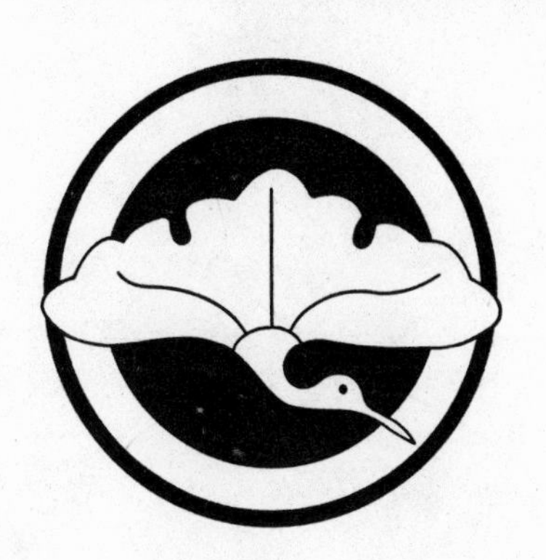

The Infertility Book

A COMPREHENSIVE MEDICAL AND EMOTIONAL GUIDE

Carla Harkness

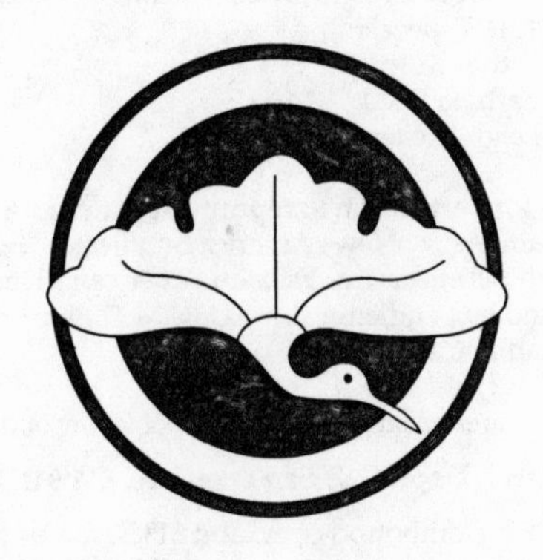

VOLCANO PRESS, INC.
SAN FRANCISCO, CALIFORNIA
VOLCANO, CALIFORNIA

Library of Congress Cataloging-in-Publication Data

Harkness, Carla, 1949–
The infertility book.

Bibliography: p.
Includes index.
1. Infertility. I. Title. [DNLM: 1. Infertility—popular works. WP 570 H282i]
RC889.H29 1986 616.6'92 87-8132
ISBN 0-912078-78-2
ISBN 0-912078-79-0 (pbk.)

We offer librarians an Alternative CIP prepared by Sanford Berman, Head Cataloger at Hennepin County Library, Edina, MN, which we believe more adequately and accurately reflects this book's scope and content.

Alternative Cataloging-in-Publication Data

Harkness, Carla, 1949–

The infertility book: a comprehensive medical and emotional guide. San Francisco, CA: Volcano Press.
PARTIAL CONTENTS: Foreword, by Robert D. Nachtigall. –Infertility experience. Self-images and social pressures. Impact on the couple. Economics of infertility. Surgery. Taking care of yourself. –Diagnosis, causes and treatment. Hormonal problems and their treatment. Endometriosis. Immunological and unexplained infertility. Pregnancy loss. New frontiers: in vitro fertilization, embryo and gamete intrafallopian tube transfers. Artificial insemination. –Resolutions. Adoption. Surrogate mothers. Child-free living. –Glossary. –Selected bibliography.

APPENDICES: Resources: medical information, referrals and emotional support. –U.S. Public Health Service regional offices.

1. Infertility. 2. Infertility—Information services—Directories. 3. "Test tube" babies. 4. Embryo transfer. 5. Artificial insemination. 6. Reproductive technology. 7. Adoption. 8. Child-free marriage. 9. Surrogate mothers. 10. Pregnancy. 11. Infertility—Economic aspects. 12. Infertility—Psychological aspects. I. Title. II. Volcano Press.
616.692

Editor:	Ruth Gottstein
Copy editor:	Loralee Windsor
Design and production:	Editorial Design/Joy Dickinson
Composition:	TBH/Typecast, Inc.
Illustrations:	Esther Kutnick
Indexer:	Barbara Roos
Project Coordinator:	Leigh Dickerson Davidson

Acknowledgment is made for permission to reprint: "A Letter to Ann Landers," reprinted with permission of Ann Landers, © News America Syndicate; "Song of Samantha," by Ronna Case, reprinted with permission of Eskaton American River Hospital; "Basal Body Temperature Chart," devised by Pendleton Tompkins, M.D., reprinted with permission of Tech-Art Publications, Arcadia, California.

Additional copies of this book are available at your local bookstore or directly from the publisher:

Volcano Press, 330 Ellis Street, Dept. INF, San Francisco, CA 94102.

Please enclose $23.50 for each clothbound copy, and $13.50 for each paperback copy ordered, which includes a charge for postage and handling. California residents please add sales tax.

Printed in the United States of America

9 8 7 6 5 4 3 2 1

CONTENTS

PART III Resolutions 215

FOREWORD

"Sarah was barren. She had no child." These terse, stark sentences appear in the eleventh chapter of Genesis, yet it was the imagination-inspiring technical wizardry of a "test-tube" baby, reflected in millions of television and magazine-cover images, that brought infertility out of the shadows of shame and into the aseptic glare of the operating room.

I am a reproductive endocrinologist, trained in both clinical skills and research, certified in two medical specialties. I have access to most of the medical knowledge and tools available for the understanding of human reproduction as we know it today. Yet I cannot help but feel that technical validation alone is neither adequate nor sufficient to the task of treating infertility. The "disease" of infertility is not experienced as an infirmity of the body, but as an unrequited longing of the human heart.

I met Carla Harkness four years ago at an infertility symposium presented by RESOLVE of Northern California. During our conversation we were struck that of the conditions for which people seek medical consultation, infertility is unique in that the "patient" is a man and a woman. We agreed that only from a shared medical and emotional perspective could two people fully sustain themselves and each other through what is viewed by most as a life crisis. This book is an effort to provide that perspective.

Infertility has no symptoms, causes no disability, and is invisible to the naked eye. It is defined in textbooks as the failure to conceive after one year of unprotected intercourse, yet in reality, infertility starts when a couple begins to fear that something may be wrong. It is the effect of this deepening apprehension that is the "disease" of infertility. Whether expressed as a melancholic wistfulness or as a life-consuming rage is individual, but feelings of anger, guilt, sadness, isolation, loneliness, frustration and remorse are universal. It is critical to understand that infertility causes stress, *not* the other way around. Even well-meaning friends and family may infuriate with suggestions to "relax," implying that your feelings are the cause of your problem, not the result. Past life decisions based upon educational, career or personal opportunities may be rehashed or ignored in the vain search for a "reason" for a dilemma which is intrinsically, inherently, and blamelessly unfair.

Time becomes the enemy. Whether it is the incessant ticking of the biologic clock, or the endlessness of waiting for the next menstrual period in a life whose pace is marked by daily temperature dots, no infertile couple accepts the passage of time with equanimity. There are unavoidable medical realities here—diagnosis is still as much art as science and treatments often require months of evaluation before they are altered or abandoned. There is no way to measure progress—you are either pregnant or not. There is no "partial credit," no "getting warmer." It is important to recognize that you will feel that things are not going well right up to the moment that you conceive.

My advice is brief. Take control of what you can. Educate yourself about what is known and what is not. Find a physician who is sufficiently experienced and interested in the treatment of infertility and establish a rational plan with defined time intervals for each step. Support your partner with as much openness as possible and seek out others who can be relied on for sympathetic and non-judgmental understanding. Recognize that the outcome is not under your control, but your choices and actions are.

Finally, take hope in the fact that the majority of you reading this book will become pregnant, and that all of you can be successful in establishing a family that satisfies the longings in your heart.

ROBERT D. NACHTIGALL, M.D.
San Francisco, California
December, 1986

ACKNOWLEDGMENTS

Realizing the dreams of both birthing my children and creating this book was a ten year effort, accomplished with the support and assistance of many people.

I would like to give special thanks and recognition to:

Robert D. Nachtigall, M.D., for devoting countless hours reviewing the medical chapters and discussing the psychological and emotional issues of infertility, for sharing his own writings, and for taking a chance on a fledgling author;

Robert P. Neff, M.D., for bringing his knowledge, steady hands, and dedicated soul to a dozen hours of meticulous surgery, and for a decade of friendship, insights, and compassion which helped me find my babies and heal my body and heart;

Cindy Renshaw, for her role in the creation of this book and living example of determination and extraordinary courage;

Nancy Whitney DeGoff, a most special, wise, and loving mom and friend, for her perspectives on loss and recovery;

Linda Palmer, for her unfailing good humor, practical suggestions, and many hours of careful editing;

Sheri Glucoft Wong, for her wisdom, compassion, and healing friendship;

Joan Hangarter, D.C., for bringing balance to my body and sharing the dream of motherhood;

Carole McGregor, for her medical research and conscientious efforts;

Alida Allison and Roberta Rosenbaum, my agents, for believing in both the subject matter and the writer and for finding the right home for my book;

Ruth Gottstein, my publisher and friend, for her commitment to birthing the best book possible, for her gentle instruction in quality writing and editing, and for her belief in miracles;

Leigh Dickerson Davidson, for her objective perspective and diligent efforts in meeting each publication deadline;

The Board of Directors and members of the Northern California Chapter of RESOLVE for their support, assistance, and written contributions to this book;

Serono Symposia, USA, for their encouragement of this project and their commitment to consumer education for the infertile;

And most important to my family—Bob, Kristen, and Baby—for their unwavering confidence, love, and patience with an often overbusy wife and mom.

I also wish to thank the following contributors and friends, along with those who wish to remain anonymous, for sharing their professional expertise and personal experiences, reviewing numerous chapter drafts, lending their voices to this text, and in many cases, for helping me through my own infertility.

Advisory Panel of Medical Specialists

David Adamson, M.D.
Assistant Clinical Professor of Obstetrics and Gynecology, Stanford University Medical Center, Palo Alto, California

Donald Galen, M.D.
Co-Director, In Vitro Fertilization Program, John Muir Hospital, Walnut Creek, California

Robert Glass, M.D.
Professor of Obstetrics and Gynecology, and Co-Director, In Vitro Fertilization Program, University of California, San Francisco

Ira Golditch, M.D.
Chief of Obstetrics and Gynecology, Kaiser Permanente Medical Center, San Francisco

Simon Henderson, M.D.
Assistant Clinical Professor of Obstetrics and Gynecology, University of California, San Francisco

Arnold Jacobson, M.D.
Founder and Co-Director, In Vitro Fertilization Program, John Muir Hospital, Walnut Creek, California

Emmett Lamb, M.D.
Professor of Obstetrics and Gynecology, University of California, San Francisco

Carl Levinson, M.D.
Professor of Obstetrics and Gynecology, University of California, San Francisco

Rose Cirelli Marques, D. Pharm.
El Camino Hospital, Mountain View, California

Alex Marques, D. Pharm.
El Camino Hospital, Mountain View, CA

Mary Martin, M.D.
Assistant Professor of Obstetrics and Gynecology and Co-Director, In Vitro Fertilization Program, University of California, San Francisco

R. Dale McClure, M.D.
Assistant Professor of Urology, University of California, San Francisco

Robert D. Nachtigall, M.D.
Associate Clinical Professor of Obstetrics and Gynecology, University of California, San Francisco

Robert P. Neff, M.D.
Assistant Professor of Obstetrics and Gynecology, University of California, San Francisco

Michael Policar, M.D.
Assistant Professor of Obstetrics and Gynecology, University of California, San Francisco

Ira Sharlip, M.D.
Assistant Clinical Professor of Urology, University of California, San Francisco

Advisory Panel on Emotional, Psychological, and Economic Issues of Infertility

Linda Applegarth, Ed.D.
Janice Chiappone, Ph.D.
Beverly Freeman, Executive Director, RESOLVE, Inc.
Joan Hangarter, D.C.
Vivian Lee, Regional Consultant for Family Planning Services, U.S. Public Health Service
Esther Levine, R.N.
Carole McGregor, R.N.
Linda Palmer, M.A.
Steve Palmer, Ph.D.
Sheri Glucoft Wong, L.C.S.W.

Advisory Panel on Legal and Psychological Issues of Adoption and Surrogate Arrangements

Philip Adams, J.D.
Jean Benward, L.C.S.W.
Nancy Whitney DeGoff, M.S.
Bonnie Gradstein, M.P.H.
Marc Gradstein, J.D.
Robert Harkness, J.D.
Diane Michelsen, M.S.W., J.D.
Halcea Valdes, M.S.W.

General Acknowledgments

Susan Adame
Carlos Alden
Becky Allen
Robert Alpert, M.A.
Teresa Roeder Alpert
Jan Antaki
Carolyn Latina Ashman
George Ashman, J.D.
Pauline Birnbaum
Josephine Berglund
Linda Brinkman
Gayle Bryant
Heather Butigan
Ken Butigan, M.A.
Cathy Cade, Ph.D.
Claire Cade
Carol Cline
Bonina Cohen, M.A.
Linda Cohen
Joseph Como
Karen Contreras, R.N.
Jean Cooley
Dandelion
Elizabeth Danner
Doris Davis
Susan Dean
Patricia Ogilvie DeGraw, R.N., B.S.N.
Bill and Norine Dolyiuk
James Donahue, Ph.D.
Sandy Duso, R.N., M.B.A.
Joan Emery, M.P.H.
Patricia Ensrud, R.N.
Elizabeth Evans, M.F.C.C.
Sharon Foley
Janica Fox
Carol Ginsburg
Patricia Hanus
Yvonne Harkness
Peggy Harrell, M.Div.
Mary J. Harrington
Ellen and Barry Hecht
Andrea Heikkinen
Esther Jakawich, R.N.
Robin Joseph
Ruth Judy, Ph.D.
Judith Webb Kay, Ph.D.
Patti LaCasse
Diann, Penelope, Mary, and Anny Lackey
Cecile Terrien Lampton, M.S.
Carol Mangravite
Karen Martin
Jan Masaoka
Charles McCoy, Ph.D.
Marjorie Casebier McCoy, D.H.L.
Linda McFadden, M.Div.
Jati McKimmie
Shan McSpadden
Phil and Judy Mullins
Jim Nishimine, M.D.
Dale Petersen
Gail and Bill Peterson
Linda Rampil, M.S.W.
Tom Renshaw
Sandy Ried
Diane Roddy
Bill Rojas
Louise Rosenbaum, Ph.D.
Carol Salzano
Cindy Salzano
Glenna Seely
Denise Nolen Shaffer
Maggie James Shepherd
Barbara Sletten
Denise Smith, R.N.
Sam Swan
Bonnie Taylor
Lana Terry
Barbara Thomson
Candy Timoney
Fred and Millie Twining
Lynn N. Villagran, MSW
Robert Williams
Donna R. Wilson
Loralee Windsor

For my Nonno Angelo,
who first saw the writer in the lonely
and frightened little girl he loved.
and
For Bob, Kristen Angela, and Baby,
who kept the faith.

INTRODUCTION

As offspring of large families my husband Bob and I had always assumed we were genetically fertile. But when we tried to conceive a child, we found to our astonishment and frustration that nature refused to cooperate. Although one unsuccessful month followed another, I refused to acknowledge my infertility and postponed seeing a specialist, stubbornly clinging to the hope that pregnancy was just a menstrual cycle away.

I finally made that appointment early in 1977–the initial step of a ten-year journey that would birth my children and heal my body and spirit. During that time I endured nearly every available female workup test, two diagnostic surgeries, two lengthy microsurgeries for endometriosis, and several years of fertility drug therapy.

Although the physical ordeal was certainly stressful–and at times debilitating–it was the emotional and psychological trauma of being infertile that terrified and nearly immobilized me. These years were spent on the "emotional roller coaster" described by so many: the cresting highs and plunging lows of hope with each ovulation, disappointment with the onset of every period, elation after each medical treatment, and despair as months and then years passed without a pregnancy. Infertility seemed to eclipse the positive parts of our lives, and we found it difficult to separate the fallout from this chronic crisis from the stresses of everyday life.

Over time Bob and I floundered as individuals and as a couple. I had a helpless, stranded feeling reminiscent of my first wilderness adventure. On that trip I was afraid I couldn't complete the unfamiliar, grueling climb and was even unsure whether I was on the right path. Sensing my fear a friend showed me the cairns–stacks of three rocks of graduated size–placed along the side of the trail. Left behind by those who had already trudged up the path, they were signs that we were headed in the right direction.

I slowly came to see infertility as a life challenge like that of the wilderness trek. To tackle this ascent I needed the cairns of medical information, emotional support, and reassurance that one does heal and move forward. I read everything I could find on the subject and joined the newly formed northern California chapter of RESOLVE, a nationwide support group for the infertile. I also attended several all-day infertility conferences, co-sponsored by RESOLVE and Serono Symposia, USA, that offered numerous workshops led by medical, legal, and mental health experts.

About three years after my initial infertility surgery, I gave birth to my first child. I thought this long-awaited and miraculous pregnancy would forever bury the anguish and self-doubt of infertility. Instead these feelings surfaced with surprising force when we tried unsuccessfully to have another child. I found myself immersed in secondary infertility, a parent of a toddler, filled with longing for another baby. Again I underwent the miserably familiar series of tests and surgeries.

Our secondary infertility lasted for nearly seven years, a time when I came to understand the feelings of the "other half": those who, after years of medical treatments, slowly concede they probably won't get pregnant. During this interval I grudgingly faced and accepted my disability, which allowed me to focus on the talents and gifts I did possess. The creation of this book was part of that transition.

I decided to write a comprehensive infertility source book that would contain a detailed, accurate summary of medical causes and treatments; a compassionate presentation of its emotional, psychological, and economic issues; and a realistic examination of options for resolution. With the encouragement of Serono Symposia, USA, and the support and assistance of national and northern California RESOLVE I began this project. I transcribed and edited the symposia proceedings and then expanded this framework with my own research and the insights of infertility patients, adoptive parents, and medical, legal, and mental health professionals.

This four-year project involved nearly a hundred women and men, each affected in some way by infertility. Sharing dozens of conversations and poignantly written histories brought moments of insight, clarity, laughter, and tears—and sometimes created healing bridges between us. I saw that those who experience this tragic reality—the infertile, their family and friends, and their physicians—often misunderstand and distrust each other. I hope this effort will provide a forum for discussion and understanding and perhaps bring some of us closer together.

From conception to birth, *The Infertility Book* has been a labor of the heart. And it seems fitting that this volume has been conceived, nurtured, labored through, and birthed by those who have been personally or professionally touched by infertility. It is a tribute to the spirit, determination, creativity, perseverance, and resilience with which they have confronted their life challenge. It is offered as a cairn for yours.

PART I

The Infertility Experience

PROLOGUE

One Woman's Story, One Man's Story

One Woman's Story

Donna grew up in the early sixties, one of five children in a happy, loving midwestern family. The eldest, Donna was given a lot of responsibility for household tasks and child care from an early age. She loved her brothers and sisters and enjoyed the company of children. As a teenager, Donna was also a favorite babysitter with many of the neighborhood kids.

She started menstruating when she was about 12. Her periods were irregular and she sometimes experienced painful premenstrual cramps. Donna's family doctor examined her but could find no physical problem. He assured her that she would bear as many children as she wanted.

Donna worked hard in high school and was awarded a scholarship to an eastern college. From a young age she had dreamed of going to college and having a career in business. She also wanted a loving marriage and several children but hoped to combine the two. She envisioned this life in her late twenties or early thirties. For now she was eager to go away to college and then begin her career.

Donna did well in college and graduated with honors. She soon found an entry level management position with a large corporation. She advanced quickly and was encouraged by her employer to work toward an MBA. She enrolled in a program at a nearby university and met Nick in one of her classes.

Both Donna and Nick were in their midtwenties, had many common interests, and were very involved with their careers and graduate studies. They dated for several months and decided to marry. During the first three years of their marriage, Donna and Nick finished their degrees and saved for a home. Believing they were fertile, they faithfully used contraceptives during this time. They were both close to 30 when they moved into their home and decided it was time to get pregnant.

Donna had read that it takes most couples six months to a year to conceive. She and Nick decided to stop using birth control and let nature take its course. Each month they hoped for a pregnancy. Donna's periods were still irregular, so they would become excited as five and sometimes six weeks passed between periods. She became so hopeful she denied the telltale signs of cramps and bloating. She requested pregnancy tests on several occasions, but all were negative.

After each anxious wait, Donna's period eventually started. When she realized she was not pregnant yet again, she would cry alone in the bathroom. Nick also felt disappointed each month but was more concerned about Donna's unhappiness and frustration.

Meanwhile Nick and Donna's friends and siblings were pregnant with their first and second children. Donna found herself jealously eyeing pregnant women on the bus. She felt angry that she was infertile and wondered why she was left out. Donna began to dread family gatherings where someone inevitably announced another pregnancy and somebody else always asked Donna what *she* was waiting for. They never approached Nick! She attended a few baby showers but found herself depressed and tearful for days afterward. Before long Donna began to decline invitations to both showers and family occasions.

After a year of unsuccessful attempts at pregnancy, Donna and Nick sought help from an infertility specialist. She felt frightened that something was wrong with her and ashamed that she had to see a physician at all. Why couldn't she "just get pregnant" like other women?

Their specialist suggested they chart Donna's basal temperature each morning and make love on alternate days around the time of ovulation. A semen analysis was done for Nick with normal results.

As the months progressed, Donna underwent a series of workup tests and became increasingly depressed and frustrated. Her sexual relationship with Nick was also noticeably affected. Their lovemaking never seemed spontaneous anymore and both of them carried a mental picture of her temperature graph. They felt under tremendous pressure and, for the first time, out of control of their lives. They argued more often, especially on the days when Donna thought she was ovulating or her period started. She felt guilty and inadequate and offered to divorce Nick so he could find a fertile woman.

Donna mentioned these problems to her specialist. He told her these were common reactions and recommended that she and Nick join an infertility support group to ease their isolation and pain. Nick was skeptical about the idea but so worried about Donna that he agreed to attend one meeting. They were both apprehensive and embarrassed when they walked into the room. As the evening went on, they were amazed and relieved to discover five other couples had similar stories and backgrounds. It was a great relief to hear others complain, laugh, and cry about the same problems. These people were loving, healthy, and well-adjusted, yet they were all experiencing fertility problems. Donna later told Nick that this was the first time in months that she didn't feel weird, abnormal, or out of place.

As the last part of her workup Donna underwent a diagnostic laparoscopy. During this surgical procedure her specialist found endometriosis on the outside of her uterus and tubes. He recommended major surgery to remove it; after this surgery, Donna and Nick will have a 50 percent chance to conceive a child.

This news was both a shock and relief to Donna. She was relieved that a medical reason had been found for their infertility. But she was shocked and angry that her body is "abnormal" and "diseased," and her chances for childbearing are only half those of other women. The surgery has been scheduled. Donna and Nick have continued meeting with their support group and are discussing the options of adoption or child-free living if she should not conceive.

Infertility has changed both Donna and Nick. They feel sadder and wiser about life but remain firmly committed to each other. Donna is tired of the emotional and medical stresses of her fertility struggle. She also worries that she and Nick may never experience pregnancy and birth. Nick is angry that Donna has had to endure the tests and still faces major surgery. He is also weary of his wife's constant unhappiness. They both worry about the high cost of infertility care and wonder why this had to happen to them.

One Man's Story

Jim was the second of three sons, an all-American boy who grew up in southern California in the late sixties. His parents encouraged their sons to excel in athletics, scouting, and academics. Jim played varsity basketball and ran cross-country in high school and college. His grades were consistently high and he was particularly drawn to electronics. Jim was popular in school, had gone steady with many girls over the years, and was sexually experienced by the time he began college.

Jim never thought much about fatherhood while growing up. Once in college he figured that if he ever did marry he'd probably want to have a couple of kids. This idea, however, was never as important as getting through school and establishing some type of career in communications.

A few years after Jim graduated from college, a mutual friend introduced him to Lisa, a high school teacher about his age. They had similar interests, hit it off immediately, and married within a year.

At first neither Jim nor Lisa wanted to have children. They had an active social life and busy careers and traveled a great deal. Lisa took birth control pills for the first eight years of their marriage and both assumed pregnancy was just a "few tries away" if they did want a child. After she turned 30, however, Lisa mentioned having a baby more often. Jim had also been thinking about fatherhood, and they agreed to quit the pill. Many of their siblings and friends were now parents, and at first they were excited about having a child of their own. After six months, however, their excitement changed to frustration. They had no luck and it seemed that someone was forever asking if they were pregnant yet.

After a year of unsuccessful tries Lisa's gynecologist suggested they begin an infertility workup. Both Jim and Lisa were dismayed by the idea that they were infertile but agreed to a few simple tests. They wanted to know if there was a problem.

A semen analysis was ordered for Jim. He balked at the idea of masturbating into a jar and having his sperm graded for quality and quantity. He knew his sex life was normal and assumed that his sperm was. Because Lisa was so insistent, he grudgingly went to the lab one day before work. With a great deal of embarrassment, he produced the sample and gave the jar to the lab technician. He went to work and tried to forget the experience.

Lisa's doctor called a few days later and asked them both to come to his office. He told them that Jim's sperm count was quite low with poor motility. He thought Jim should see a urologist for further evaluation before Lisa underwent any invasive fertility tests. They were both stunned by the news and couldn't think of much to say. They wrote down the name of the urologist and left the office.

They drove home in silence. Jim's thoughts flickered with images of basketball games, school dances, and past sexual encounters. He remembered sweating out a couple of passionate evenings where no one had bothered about contraceptives. He couldn't believe he wasn't fertile. He wondered if he would eventually become impotent.

When they got home, Lisa tried to talk about the visit but he angrily told her to leave him alone. They agreed to see the urologist the following week and drop the subject until then. They somehow got through the next few days. On a few occasions Lisa tried to touch or hold Jim, but he brushed her away.

They went to the urologist's office at the scheduled time. Lisa was close to tears and Jim was frightened. The doctor interviewed them in his office and then gave Jim a thorough physical examination. He found a varicocele of the left scrotum that he said might be contributing to the problem. He also asked Jim to produce another semen sample so he could personally evaluate it. He suggested Jim and Lisa return in two days to assess the situation.

When they got home, Jim could hardly face Lisa. He was scared, ashamed, and for the first time in their relationship, felt inadequate. Maybe she would leave him. Lisa was both worried about Jim and frightened that she would not bear a child. She tried to console him, suggesting that the urologist might help them. Jim angrily told her to leave him alone and go find a fertile man; she could have a divorce anytime she wanted. It was one of their worst arguments. Lisa left the house in tears and returned late that evening. Jim pretended he was asleep.

On their next visit the urologist confirmed the low sperm count and poor motility problem. With no treatment at all he said they had roughly a 25 percent chance for a spontaneous pregnancy. With treatment their chances for pregnancy might increase to 30 to 50 percent providing Lisa did not have any fertility problems. He offered to review the medical and surgical alternatives in detail, now or at a later appointment. He also told them about the options of artificial insemination by donor, adoption, and child-free living and urged the couple to call anytime with questions or concerns. He also recommended they seek emotional support.

Both Jim and Lisa were devastated by the news. At best they seemed to have a 50 percent chance to have a child. In reality their odds were probably less than that. Once they were home, Jim stated that he didn't want to have surgery or adopt and he certainly didn't want another guy's sperm inseminated in Lisa! She was furious with him. She'd certainly have surgery or take fertility drugs if *she* had a problem!

Lisa now seemed obsessed about having a baby. Jim reminded her that she had put it off for eight years. Why was it such a big deal now? Why couldn't she drop it and take what life gave them? They could travel, sleep late every weekend, buy a new car.

Another week of hostile, bitter exchanges followed. After yet another horrible argument, Lisa tearfully told Jim she loved him but couldn't go on this way. She thought they needed professional help, as well as emotional support. She suggested they see a therapist experienced in fertility problems, tell their friends and families about the situation, and check out an infertility support group. Jim, too, wanted to save their marriage. He agreed to this course of action.

Their families had mixed reactions to the news. Lisa's mother and Jim's sister had lost several pregnancies and were sympathetic and supportive. Jim's parents, however, seemed defensive and embarrassed by the news. His friends weren't exactly helpful either. "I'd be happy to stand in for you, buddy!" and "Shooting blanks, huh, Jim?" were a couple of responses. For the first time in his life Jim felt abnormal and sadly alone.

When they attended their first support group meeting, Jim sat in a distant corner of the living room. He still couldn't identify with infertile people. Jim didn't talk much but listened carefully. Several of the men also had low sperm counts and the couples were experiencing the same marital and self-esteem problems as he and Lisa. Some of the women complained that their husbands "didn't care" about their infertility problem. It dawned on Jim that men have been culturally conditioned to work, compete, provide, and, to a certain extent, hide their emotions. He saw that he wasn't alone and began to look forward to the meetings.

Lisa and Jim also sought counseling from a professional therapist. In weekly sessions they are now clarifying their feelings about having a child and examining the options available to them.

Despite this support infertility is a difficult burden to shoulder. Jim and Lisa are painfully aware that many other couples conceive easily, some of their friends and relatives still offer endless advice, and they still wonder, "Why us?"

CHAPTER 1

Self-Images and Social Pressures

► *I have always been an avid reader of history. Barrenness has been a curse and stigma in every society I've studied. In my own ethnic heritage it is the worst thing that can happen to a woman. Small wonder I felt the doom of the ages when I learned of my own infertility.*

► *The last straw came at a Christmas party in a home filled with small children. While my husband held an infant, someone loudly remarked, "Oh doesn't he look so natural holding that baby? He ought to be a daddy!"*

I walked outside and sat in the dark. Waves of hate washed over me both toward them and myself. Why doesn't my body work right? Why can't people think before they speak? Why do their thoughtless remarks still hurt?

Human beings have been mating and, with varying degrees of success, reproducing for millions of years. Although billions of babies have been born, countless couples have also encountered fertility problems or pregnancy loss throughout the ages. This is because nature has endowed both females and males with delicately balanced, complex reproductive systems. The slightest obstruction, imbalance, or abnormality can disrupt the intricate harmony of the chemical processes necessary for sperm production, ovulation, fertilization, implantation, and pregnancy to occur.

Still, we live on a crowded planet, surrounded by fertile humans, fauna, and flora. As a result, many people tend to take fertility for granted, assuming they can plan or control childbearing. Although most couples do achieve a pregnancy within a year of unprotected intercourse, about 10 million Americans experience fertility problems at any given time. For these women and men, a successful pregnancy may be an unattainable goal.

The Social Pressures of Infertility

For millenia it was essential for humans to multiply lest the species die out. Although the earth is now a dangerously crowded planet, that value persists and is encountered by both infertile women and men and couples who are voluntarily childless. The social pressure to bear a child is usually conveyed by family and friends, and these relationships often become painful and strained.

► *I think my relationship with my mother has suffered the most. I have felt inadequate and ashamed to discuss my infertility with her. When my younger sister had her babies, I felt myself drift away from all of them. They couldn't understand my feelings and it was less painful to avoid their company.*

In a society where few are bold enough to ask your annual income, nearly everyone will inquire about your fertility. If a couple does not produce a child within a "reasonable length of time," their friends and relatives usually ask why. Remarks and questions may range from the subtle ("You two sure would make great parents!") to the guilt-provoking ("I'm just dying to be a grandmother!") to the downright cruel ("What's wrong with you two?" "Just relax, you're trying too hard." "Don't you know how to do it?" "When are you going to stop shooting blanks?").

This external pressure on the infertile couple is further intensified by specific occasions and social situations that celebrate pregnancy, children, and the extended family: holidays, other women's pregnancies, and baby showers.

► *Christmas was the pinnacle of pain, especially the year our nephew was born on Christmas Eve. Everyone raved about how much he looked like my husband. I'll always remember the way my husband wept in my arms that night. Seven years of his being strong for me finally ended in an emotional release for him.*

Throughout the year holidays bring almost monthly reminders of our infertility. Mother's Day and Father's Day, Halloween, Passover, Easter, Thanksgiving, Chanukah, and Christmas are largely centered around children. You may have fantasized for years about how to celebrate these occasions with your child.

Christmas and Chanukah are probably the most difficult holidays for the infertile. Store windows are filled with toys and adorable tots line up to visit Santa. Cards arrive from smiling and perhaps growing families, along with invitations to family reunions and holiday parties. These gatherings usually involve contact with children and infants, and the merriment and refreshments encourage remarks and discussion of your fertility.

And when you long for a baby, jealousy and anger toward pregnant women are natural reactions; it is difficult not to stare at their bulging bellies with frustration. Seeing someone else's body swell with child can hurt deeply.

► *My feelings were very intense and on occasion the thought of being around a pregnant friend would reduce me to hysterical crying.*

It often seems as if everyone you know is expecting. The pregnancies of close friends and relatives are especially painful and often evoke ambivalent feelings. You may feel genuine happiness for their good fortune yet dread socializing with them, fearing your own reactions as well as pity or insensitivity from others.

These painful feelings are exacerbated by the inevitable baby shower invitations. These gatherings often epitomize an infertile woman's isolation.

► *I wished I would never have to suffer my hysteria after yet another baby shower. Finally, I stopped going. I could no longer deal with my feelings.*

She must sit in a room filled with women—most of whom are already mothers or perhaps also expecting—and watch an extremely pregnant friend open gifts of cute baby things. Her infertility either goes unnoticed or, even worse, is acknowledged in pitying glances. Back home she may cry for hours or even days afterward, wondering for the thousandth time "Why me? What did I do to deserve this?" Her husband is often unable to console her and may experience similar feelings on occasions like Christmas or Father's Day. (Chapter 7 includes suggestions for coping with these social events along with a discussion of the unique pressures encountered by infertile stepparents and single women.)

The Emotional Fallout of Infertility

► *Infertility is a silent tragedy. How do you explain to someone that you had a rough night because there was no baby to keep you awake, that your house is too clean and there are no toys cluttering the floor? Would anyone understand that you have cried over Pampers commercials?*

Although 10 million face this problem each infertile individual usually feels isolated and alone, largely because this is an invisible affliction. Without asking we can't tell who has shared our experience and, until recently, infertility has rarely been discussed or acknowledged. Many couples are still reluctant to reveal their problem to friends or relatives.

The 1980s are a particularly painful decade in which to be infertile. The post–World War II baby boomers are now producing a boomlet of their own, and the current wave of maternity fashions, natural birthing classes, infant carriers, and breast-feeding debates emphasizes an infertile couple's isolation and loneliness. "I felt I was being excluded from some magic parent's club," one woman remarked. "It was as if everyone had been asked to dance but me." Many temporarily withdraw from the world of children while they struggle with their infertility.

Altered Self-Images

► *Everywhere I looked I saw pregnant women. I felt conspicuously infertile. The high following my surgery faded into depression and disgust with my body when I again failed to conceive.*

"I'm no good," I'd fume. "It must be a curse. Other women can do it easily. What's wrong with me?"

Many infertile women and men feel disappointment or disgust with their bodies. Often premenstrual cramps and fullness bring on tears and intense feelings of failure for a woman, and she may feel her body is defective on these days. Long-term infertility can also make a man feel inadequate and undermine his sense of masculinity.

Old childhood insecurities and feelings of inferiority often resurface. Once again we feel odd or that we don't belong. Back in high school we may have yearned for blonde hair, a perfect figure, or athletic prowess. Now it is the ability to conceive after 6 to 12 months of unprotected intercourse. Strong self-images that took years to develop often weaken.

Understandably sexuality can also be affected. We may feel physically unattractive or associate sex solely with procreation. The goals of pregnancy and pleasure become fused, and the failure to realize the former often affects the latter.

Guilt Feelings

► *It's Thanksgiving and I cry again. Mourning my unborn child, not knowing if he would have my husband's curly hair or my big round eyes. What have I done in my past not to be able to do such a simple thing as make a baby?*

► *I remembered hushed conversations I wasn't supposed to hear as a child. A "barren" woman would be discussed in pitying voices amidst speculation of what was wrong with her. As our infertility dragged on, I became more fearful and defensive. I started to think that I was being punished.*

Many search for a reason *why* they are infertile. They wonder if this is punishment for being "bad" and undeserving of happiness or retribution for past "offenses," such as an abortion, a miscarriage greeted with relief, or premarital sex. Religious training can reinforce such thinking; some try to atone for past wrongs and regard painful or embarrassing workup tests and surgeries as part of their punishment.

An infertile partner often feels guilty for causing the problem, thinking: "It's all my fault," or "If she was with someone else, she could get pregnant." To compensate for this inadequacy, either or both partners may try to keep the relationship perfect in other ways or conversely may seek other sexual partners.

Loss of Control

► *Two days ago my period came again. We tried so hard this month, timing our intimacy to create a new life. We, who try to control everything in our lives so perfectly. Do we try again and again? When do we, or should we, give up? We feel as if our lives are on hold.*

For anyone who wishes to plan childbearing, rather than just "let it happen," infertility is a frustrating turn of events. Successful, self-confident individuals and "over-achievers" can be particularly devastated by this problem. After reaching other goals, they are unable to perform the "simple" biological feat of a successful pregnancy. In reality, of course, fertility is *not* easily managed or controlled!

A long-term fertility problem often creates a state of limbo for both partners. They don't know whether they'll have the child they want, how long to pursue treatment, whether adoption or child-free living is an appropriate option, or even if their marriage can withstand this crisis. Women especially may defer career moves or advanced studies until their infertility is resolved. It may also be difficult to make mutual decisions about occupation changes, job relocation, and financial investments during this time.

Resentment

► *My younger brother and his wife called to say they were expecting a child and it was a "surprise." We had invested many years and dollars in charts, drugs, and surgeries to no avail. It wasn't hard to imagine the pity the rest of the family would direct toward infertile me. It was so unfair.*

Media reports of unwanted pregnancies and tragic instances of child abuse are ironic realities to the infertile. Eager to parent, they endure any number of medical procedures and untold emotional stress in their desperation to have a child.

Unfortunately the ability to reproduce is not related to goodness or whether one deserves to have a child. Conceiving and bearing a healthy child is largely a matter of luck and genetics. Like other victims of disease or misfortune, the infertile are simply unlucky.

Psychological Stages of Infertility

Infertility is often described as a "life crisis," a time of both internal turmoil and external pressure. Many women and men pass through several psychological stages of confrontation and acceptance. They also experience complex feelings of loss: of the joyous event of "just getting pregnant" without medical testing or treatment, of control over the ability to plan reproduction, and to some extent, one's life. For some infertility becomes an obsession and a symbol of their failure to meet personal as well as cultural expectations.

Many health professionals apply one of two models, or a combination of both, to describe and facilitate the coping process of infertility. The Kübler-Ross/Menning model suggests a finality of psychological acceptance after several stages of denial, anger, and grief. The chronic coping model suggested by Drs. Jeanne Fleming and Kenneth Burry likens infertility to a protracted process, and for some people, a lifelong reality.

Kübler-Ross/Menning Model

Elisabeth Kübler-Ross in her landmark work, *On Death and Dying*, identified transitional stages that individuals experience when facing their own death. Barbara Eck Menning, a nurse and founder of RESOLVE (a support organization described at the end of this chapter), has applied Ross's theory to the infertility challenge. Like those confronting death, Menning suggests, the infertile individual or couple passes through similar stages during the struggle for acceptance and resolution. This is not a linear process; each partner will probably move through these stages at different paces, and either may periodically regress to a previous phase.

► *Infertile. Not me. Maybe next month I'll get pregnant and this will all have been a bad dream. Seeking help would make the infertility real.*

Denial or surprise is a common initial reaction, perhaps after years of avoiding pregnancy, to a diagnosis of infertility. Believing you had been controlling reproduction, you suddenly discover it is elusive or even unattainable. This denial serves an important psychological purpose. It gives us time to absorb and process distressing news before pursuing a course of action.

Denial gives way to anger or rage toward life in general, at God, the cosmos or fate, or, more specifically, toward your infertile spouse, physician, or fertile friends and coworkers.

► *I was busy withdrawing from friends who were having their second children while I was having my second operation. This time major surgery determined and possibly corrected the cause. My chances of conceiving weren't good, but I was ecstatic and once again full of hope. I began to bargain with God for a pregnancy.*

No results. In my subsequent anger I began questioning the existence of God. Was He not listening or just not there? How could I deal with all my anger?

This anger may also be tinged with feelings of envy, frustration, powerlessness, or resentment of this injustice. In some cases infertile women and men may seek other sexual partners to "punish" their mates and reaffirm their own desirability.

Anger may also be vented inward in the form of depression. You may feel victimized and out of control. Symptoms include apathy, insomnia, lethargy, a marked increase or decrease of appetite, crying spells, anxiety, and feelings of hopelessness or despair. Long-term infertility can become an obsession or the central focus of life.

A period of grief, either for your present infertility or for the baby you will never birth, commonly follows anger or depression.

► *I finally let loose. The pain, hurt, and guilt screamed their way out. I was immobilized and cried for three days. As I sobbed in my husband's embrace, I wondered why this was happening to us.*

► *My daughter is 14 months old. I gave birth to her and yet I feel like crying now just remembering the intense pain at thinking I would never become pregnant. Not ever being able to have a baby—or at least experiencing the possibility of that—calls for intense grieving, as if you have lost a child.*

The duration and intensity of mourning depends on whether infertility is long-term or permanent, as well as on individual temperament. Most people report periods of grief lasting a few months to a year, although medical treatments and just plain hoping may continue indefinitely. Some carry this pain far into old age and are moved to tears at the mention of their infertility or miscarriage of three or four decades ago.

Our society does not acknowledge infertility as an occasion for mourning, and at first we too may not recognize grief as it occurs. While women often release grief through tears, because of cultural conditioning men often bury pain until it erupts in some other way. In any case going through the motions of everyday life and interacting with family and friends can seem an overwhelming burden.

Each individual and couple grieves in a private way—some by crying alone or sharing their feelings with close friends, others by writing poetry or creating rites of passage.

► *Sarah and I had dreamed of a biological child for years and had accumulated booties, rattles, and other gifts. After years of medical treatments, we finally decided it was time to pursue adoption. To release our grief, we buried the gifts in the backyard. We feel this ritual marked a passage in our lives and created a place to hold our grief. Now we can search for our adopted child with a new love and enthusiasm.*

You must finish the grieving process before acceptance of infertility can occur. While this seems to last forever, it does gradually diminish. You probably won't forget your infertility, but memories will be fleeting rather than daily obsessions.

► *While I awaited surgery, I slowly began to accept my infertility. This stage was not as bad as waiting for the diagnosis. I began to see myself as unique and special for experiencing something that not everyone does. The pain of infertility, even intractable infertility like mine, can be a stepping stone to greater insight and compassion for the human experience.*

Infertility has changed me forever and no one will ever care about it as much as I do. Everyone must resolve it his or her own way. You are alone in this, as at death. Others can support and talk with you, but you yourself must come to terms with it and finally face the fertile world again.

Accepting your infertility is the first step toward resolution. "Resolving" is a complex concept that includes acceptance of infertility and a healing from its losses, followed by a desire to pursue an appropriate option such as adoption, continued medical treatment, or child-free living. At this stage a resurgence of energy and self-esteem usually occurs.

Chronic Coping Model

► *Infertility has been a part of my life for nine years now. Some days it weighs more heavily than others. But it's there every day. I haven't really reached acceptance that this has happened to me, but I have learned to live with it.*

Jeanne Fleming, Ph.D., and Kenneth Burry, M.D., among other health professionals, suggest that many couples view infertility as a chronic problem. For example, those with mild or moderate fertility problems often have endless hope of achieving a pregnancy during their reproductive years. Others may encounter unexplained or secondary infertility or may embark on a medical or surgical treatment that has a fairly good success rate and creates new hope for pregnancy. But after months or years of continued infertility, some become chronically depressed or immobilized by the problem, like those coping with a handicapped child, troubled marriage, or a loved one who has run away or disappeared. Couples caught in this chronic model often avoid poignant reminders of their infertility, which they describe as a "lifelong reality" they are unable to accept or resolve.

Fleming and Burry suggest that these couples should approach their infertility in two ways:

- Decide whether and how they will parent by clarifying their attitudes toward adoption and child-free living
- Develop appropriate ways to cope with their long-term problem

The latter strategy involves acknowledging each partner's feelings, rebuilding confidence and self-esteem through other goals and achievements, and finding emotional support.

Tools for Meeting the Challenge

► *You can reach out and look for those special people who can say, "I understand. I've been there too." There were times when I clung like a drowning woman to people who let me. And when my head was high enough above water to have some perspective, I tried to be there for those who were sinking.*

For years there were few sources of emotional support for the infertile. Fortunately this is no longer true; you need not face this problem alone. Many have found vast relief just hearing someone else verbalize their anger and heartache. Reading about the struggles and triumphs of others, or speaking to them by phone or in support groups, can provide inspiration and a much needed reality check. Some specialists encourage such dialogue and will, upon request, introduce their patients to others in the same situation.

Support Groups

► *Talking about infertility has helped us cope, and being part of a support group put infertility into perspective. No one should be afraid of a support group. Sometimes you cry, but there's lots of laughter too!*

Many people are hesitant about joining an infertility support group. Some even think seeking such help is an admission of emotional instability. Therapists and psychologists, however, agree that the intense and often overwhelming emotions associated with infertility are a natural reaction to a real crisis.

Support groups are a safe refuge from a fertile world, where one can express feelings and receive empathy and understanding. The groups focus *solely* on the feelings and problems of infertility, so other personal issues are not addressed. This setting can provide valuable coping suggestions and moral support.

While a support group can't guarantee a pregnancy, it can ease some of the pain and isolation of infertility. Many couples find it a useful vehicle to examine their feelings and options for resolutions.

► *One of the women in our group brought her newborn adopted baby to our meeting. It was incredible: We passed the baby around, and for many of us, it was the first time in years we'd been able to hold and touch a baby without terrible pain. It was as if this baby was a symbol not only of what we could ourselves have one day if we wished, but also of all the sorrow we'd gone through. We felt so close to each other that night and went home feel-*

ing as if we'd been touched by something really miraculous, having been able to open ourselves up to our feelings instead of shutting down for protection.

A feeling of unity often develops in support groups as couples move toward resolution, and lifelong friends are sometimes made in the process!

Professional Counseling

► *After seven years of infertility we decided to consult a therapist. It was the best thing we ever did. With her help we were able to separate the effects of our infertility from other personal and marital problems. We finished our therapy feeling better about ourselves and deeply committed to each other.*

Some individuals or couples are reluctant to confide in new acquaintances or feel awkward in a support group setting. If feelings of depression or inadequacy persist, a consultation with a therapist experienced with fertility issues may be helpful. Because infertility often raises old insecurities, it is important to separate the misfortune of this problem from such notions as punishment or inferiority.

RESOLVE

RESOLVE is a nonprofit organization founded in 1973 by Barbara Eck Menning, a nurse who had personally experienced infertility. Unable to find emotional support, Menning began the first RESOLVE group in Boston. For many years she devoted her energy to providing medical information, emotional support, and referrals to infertile women and men, as well as to the medical community. Today RESOLVE, Inc., has grown to a national office and 45 affiliated chapters within the United States—many of which offer monthly meetings, support groups, adoption information, phone counseling, medical referrals, and newsletters—and, with Serono Symposia, USA, cosponsors numerous all-day informational conferences. Throughout this book, the reader is referred to this important ally for both the infertile and concerned health professionals.

The infertility struggle, focused both within and without, is a rocky passage with an uncertain outcome. It also raises painful and difficult questions. Do we expect ourselves to produce a biological child at any physical, emotional, or financial cost? How do we assess available medical treatments? Are adoption or child-free living acceptable alternatives to our extended families and ourselves? How can we keep ourselves and our marriages intact while searching for an appropriate resolution? In their own time, each couple or individual must find their own answers to these questions.

An infertility experience also affords an opportunity for personal growth and triumph. By confronting the problem, weathering its challenges, and learning to cope as individuals and partners, you can emerge as healthy, loving, and fulfilled people. The following chapters offer information, personal insights, and coping suggestions for this difficult task.

CHAPTER 2

Impact on the Couple

► *Bill and I have been married for 17 years and I have never been pregnant. Back in our early marriage I had a very strong desire to have a baby. Nothing ever happened. We decided to go through many procedures including numerous sperm counts, laparoscopy, and artificial insemination by donor. It was a tremendous strain on our marriage. I was always depressed, felt like a failure, and hated to be around baby things. I wondered, "Why me? Why am I so different? What's wrong with me?" I felt abandoned by my friends and not understood, even by my husband.*

► *Infertility was a great sorting out of our relationship with two results: we wanted to be married and felt a strong need to be parents. We both agree that, if this is the problem we were dealt in the game of life, we'll take it and run!*

A fertility problem, usually detected within the first decade of marriage, may be a couple's first major adversity. For many, infertility appears after other life goals have been carefully planned and successfully realized. Unlike other problems, however, infertility does not always respond to rational planning, thoughtful analysis, or short-term crisis strategy. In fact a couple may face the emotional turmoil of tests, surgeries, or medical treatments with no guarantee of success.

Increasing numbers of couples who have waited until their mid- or late thirties to try for a pregnancy are experiencing fertility problems. Some have deferred pregnancy until careers or financial stability were established. Others have embarked on second or third marriages and are anxious to become pregnant right away. Marriages in which one mate is considerably older than the other may also encounter difficulties. For all these couples the pressure of a ticking biological clock magnifies the other stresses of infertility.

In any case, just as having too many children too soon can tax a marriage, infertility takes its toll. Problems with differing cultural perspectives, communication, and sexuality often arise unexpectedly and sometimes simultaneously. Even stable, loving marriages of five or ten years can be strained by these new challenges and dilemmas. This painful period of adjustment and growth, however, can also be an opportunity to enhance and deepen commitment as lovers and partners.

Men's and Women's Perspective on Infertility

Because of their cultural conditioning and ethnic heritage, women and men often bring very different perspectives to an infertility problem. As pressures build, each mate may be unable to understand the other's reactions, and couples often drift apart. An open discussion of each partner's point of view can improve communication. Recognizing their differences, they can once again understand and support each other.

Dr. Janice Chiappone, a northern California psychologist, recently studied the responses of several hundred infertile men and women through personal interviews and questionnaires. She concludes that infertility affects women's lives to a larger extent than men's and has a significantly greater effect on a woman's self-image and feelings about marriage, sexuality, and career.

Chiappone suggests that bearing and raising a child is intricately tied to a woman's self-concept. Because of cultural conditioning and ethnic background many women define an essential part of their identity through the relationships of marriage and motherhood. Even in the United States, many ethnic cultures grant women status primarily through these achievements. From the time they are little girls, most females are taught that women become mothers through pregnancy. Adoption is rarely mentioned in some cultures and may actually be considered a stigma. Thus when the prospect of biological motherhood is threatened or unattainable, women feel bitter disappointment and anger.

Conversely, our society largely defines a man's identity through his work or occupation. Although saddened by an inability to sire a child and the subsequent loss of genetic lineage, men usually don't dwell as long on the issue. And, unlike women, men do not lose the physical experience of pregnancy and birth.

Women may also think and talk more about infertility because they, more than their husbands, receive the questions and comments of curious relatives and friends. Even when the man is the infertile partner, he is rarely asked about the couple's child-free life-style.

Finally, a woman often feels more isolated by infertility. Those oriented to the traditional roles of wife and mother, without educational or career accomplishments to offset the absence of children, are often unable to find support from friends and family busy bearing and raising their own children.

Women who have already attained educational or career goals and wish to plan and time their pregnancies are often surprised and isolated when a fertility problem occurs. They may encounter several reactions from family and friends, including criticism for waiting too long while pursuing "selfish" goals and comments about their obsession with becoming pregnant should they opt for drug or surgery treatment. Neither response provides understanding or emotional support.

Communication

► *We would often lie awake at night and talk about being childless. I felt terribly guilty that I had the physical problem.*

"If he had chosen someone else," I would think, "he would be a father right now."

We went around in terrible circles.

"I know you really want kids and you're not having them with me." I would shakily initiate the argument.

"Yes, I'd like to be a father. But you're more important to me than fatherhood."

"Great choice! Me or your kids. You could have both with someone else."

"I don't want somebody else. I want you."

So it would go. We'd drop the subject for a few weeks and then it would start all over again, usually when a period marked another month's failure.

Infertility is usually a time of unrelenting stress for the couple. Besides meeting the daily challenges of life they must make important decisions about fertility testing, medication, possible surgery, or alternatives to biological birth. Often resentments surface and tempers flare under such pressure. It may become increasingly difficult for a couple to communicate their feelings or make important decisions together.

Guilt and anger are common reactions to infertility. When a medical problem is found in only one partner, she or he may feel solely responsible for and guilty about the situation. Miscarriages can also evoke guilt, as can past abortions and imagined "sins" or transgressions.

Taking Responsibility

► *My ex-husband called my infertility "the greatest tragedy of* his *life." He wanted me to try all available medical treatments. I was cautious and fearful of more surgery and drugs. This, along with other problems, destroyed our marriage.*

Couples sometimes disagree over which, if any, course of medical treatment to pursue. Sometimes one partner wants to proceed quickly with testing, surgery, or perhaps drug therapy, while the other wants to move slowly. A frank discussion with your physician about recommended procedures and drugs, along with peer or professional counseling, can help you both decide on the best course of treatment.

Mates also commonly argue over who should take responsibility for the many details of the treatment and resolution process. Often the woman feels she is shouldering too much of the struggle: scheduling doctor appointments, studying medical literature, following up on adoption leads, and so on. If her spouse assumes a passive role, she may resent spending so much of *her* time dealing with *their* problem. The burden is compounded if she is also confronting a medical problem.

Many couples ease this pressure by dividing the tasks and giving each partner some responsibility. For example, the man might schedule medical appointments and research relevant infertility literature. The woman might follow up on adoption leads and contact support organizations.

Expressing Emotion

► *My husband waited until this year even to admit our problem. I think back to my son's infancy as a happy time of life, one in which I thought I was normal. After all I had a baby I didn't try to conceive. Little did I know he was to be my first and last. I went through the entire range of feelings from denial to anger to depression and tears. I have been waiting at the point of acceptance for my husband. He faulted me for a lack of faith and effort during these past three years. As a result I have not shared a lot of the pain that I felt. Now my husband is reaching acceptance that we will have no more biological children. I hurt for him because I know how he feels.*

Venting feelings is another common communication problem. Although both mates find that infertility is a trying time, they may cope in different ways. In many cases partners move through the emotional phases of infertility at different paces and one may reach acceptance while the other feels chronically depressed or angry. Cultural conditioning can surface in their behavior: While a man often buries his anger in painful silence, his wife may cry or vocalize hers frequently to doctors, counselors, or friends willing to listen.

Some women complain that their partners "tune out" when they express their feelings: "He just doesn't care about our infertility!" Many men, on the other hand, feel overwhelmed by endless infertility conversations and tears: "She can't stop talking about it!" Other men, aware of their wives' physical and emotional pain, try to spare them additional grief by holding in their own anger.

Merle Bombardieri, a clinical social worker, has suggested a "20-minute rule" for infertility discussions between mates. This time is equally divided between the partners. After the time is up, the subject may not be discussed again until the next scheduled conversation. This way time is created for both discussion and diversion, and both partners feel their needs are met.

Keeping the lines of communication open is critical during an infertility struggle. Some couples find that joining a support group provides a perspective on their problems and fosters understanding between them; others derive solace through speaking with another infertile person or with a trusted friend or relative. If communication problems persist, however, consider professional counseling.

Sexuality

► *When my temperature fell a few tenths of a degree and then rose the next day, we would enter "egg night syndrome." There would be a scheduled atmosphere to sex. At first we would joke about command performances, but before long the humor faded.*

We would both become anxious. I would expect him to "deliver" and worry he would be too tired or upset to have sex. He would feel the pressure of that expectation and resent being forced to perform. We later realized, after many heated arguments, that as a man and woman, we approached this situation from very different perspectives.

As a woman, I felt I was carrying the medical burden of infertility. I was going for monthly checkups, facing possible surgery, and taking my temperature daily. All he had to do was deliver his sperm at the right time of the month.

He told me he resented my assumption that he could perform at will. The tension increased as the months passed. We found ourselves arguing more often around that time of the cycle.

Infertility's emotional roller coaster of hope and despair will undoubtedly affect a couple's sex life. Along with the pressure to have sex "every other day around ovulation," there is anger and frustration when menstruation marks another month's disappointment. Low self-esteem and feelings of inadequacy and guilt often become tied to sexual performance. In this negative atmosphere past sexual problems can resurface. At a time when each partner most needs special understanding, tenderness and intimacy, they may in fact drift apart, argue more often, and resent each other.

After repeated, methodical attempts to conceive, lovemaking often becomes mechanical and scheduled. It's common to feel self-conscious and obsessed with "successful sex"—erection and ejaculation of semen into the vagina. The couple's orientation changes from pleasure to reproduction, and sex may seem more like a duty.

Both partners may now focus on the woman as a receptacle for sperm, and her pleasure may be ignored. Similarly the male may be expected to deliver his semen on call (either in the bedroom or at the lab or doctor's office for tests or inseminations), with scant attention to arousal and foreplay. Thus there may be little concern for the sexual feelings of either mate.

If infertility persists, lovemaking may actually become associated with failure, and either partner may feel sexually undesirable or inadequate. In some cases one or both may seek other sexual partners in an effort to reaffirm their desirability or perhaps even punish themselves or their mate.

That infertility will affect your intimacy seems just as inevitable as scheduling lovemaking on your optimal fertile days. To counteract and alleviate this stress:

- Discuss your sexual concerns at a time when you are most relaxed and won't be interrupted. Your infertility poses many obstacles to spontaneous and healthy sex. This is a chance to communicate openly and improve your sexual relationship.

- Consider forgoing temperature charting after a month or two; or, if you continue graphing, take turns recording temperatures and initiating lovemaking on fertile days. The BBT chart often becomes an obsession. Before long, you may find yourselves making love only on Days 10, 12, and 14 of the cycle! Some couples, who find that the wife has become the "sex dictator," assign temperature charting to the husband. It can be an enormous relief to share this responsibility with your partner, and it may rekindle your sex life!

- Think of sex as an expression of love *throughout the month*, rather than associating it solely with reproduction. Be spontaneous as often as possible and take time to please and arouse each other. Extend foreplay and tell your partner what pleases and excites you: Experiment and heighten your sexual pleasure.

- Be realistic about the effects of infertility on your sex life. Don't expect the earth to move every month around ovulation time or insist on making love if your partner feels tired or uncomfortable. Remember that touching and holding each other are also important expressions of love. Genuine respect and consideration of your mate's feelings should be more important than achieving pregnancy this cycle. Gentleness and understanding now can prevent long-term sexual problems.

- Remember that even long-term infertility is still a brief time window in your sexual relationship. Before you decided to get pregnant, pleasure was the sole focus of your sexuality. This will again be true after you have resolved your infertility or completed your childbearing.

- If permanent infertility is diagnosed, expect a grieving period when sex will be difficult or unappealing. As you both heal over time, your intimacy can become deeper and stronger.

If your sexual problems do not improve, discuss the situation with your specialist. Try not to feel embarrassed: Sexual problems are common among infertile couples and physicians frequently hear such complaints. Your doctor can refer you to a therapist trained in sexual counseling. Seeking assistance now can prevent long-term difficulties.

Coping: A Celebration of the Couple

Fertility in itself does not guarantee a loving, lifelong marriage. The divorce courts are filled with couples who had no problem at all reproducing. It is tempting to assume that "if we could only have a baby, we'd live happily ever after," but those who have birthed a child after infertility can affirm that marital stress continues after parenthood.

It is easy to forget that first and foremost you are lovers. It was passion, respect, and love that brought you together long before you knew about infertility. You began your family as a couple, and regardless of whether you have children, you hope to greet old age as a twosome.

Infertility can create a time for reflection on your goals as a couple and as individuals. You can use this challenge to renew and strengthen your commitment. Carol Salzano, former president of the northern California chapter of RESOLVE, writes:

February is great! There are no holiday cartoon specials, Halloween goblins, store Santas, Easter baskets, or other painful reminders of what each of us is striving to achieve. Once a year this 28-day month (the perfect cycle) ushers us from winter into spring. This is a month to celebrate!

Sometimes we are so obsessed with the infertility struggle that we forget ourselves as a couple. Tension begins to rule our relationship and cloud our feelings for each other. February is the month to put our struggles aside for a moment and reflect upon what it is to be a couple again; those two people who met, fell in love, and made a commitment.

Valentine's Day, with its traditional flowers, candy hearts, and cupids symbolizes that love. This day should be enjoyed just for its romance. Let this day be your holiday to reinforce the romance in your marriage.

Have fun, laugh, and enjoy yourselves! Most importantly, celebrate that the two of you are already a family. May this brief renewal bring added strength to face the future and what it may hold.

Try to make every month a February! Renew your commitment to that special person with whom you share your life. Playing the "What if?" game may help. What if you had all the children you wanted right now? What new goals would you set? How would you relate to each other, please each other sexually and romantically? Why not start right now?

You deserve a lot of credit for weathering this together. Treat yourselves to many pleasurable rewards during this trying time, and remember the ancient saying, "This, too, shall pass." If dealt with in a healthy and positive way, the infertility experience can strengthen the bond between you.

CHAPTER 3

The Economics of Infertility

► *We found the financial strain of infertility just as difficult as all of the emotional pressure. Since our treatment went on for five years and required several surgeries, months of fertility drug treatment, and numerous office procedures, the bills were considerable. Even with medical insurance our portion was staggering. A large percentage of my paycheck went toward these costs. There just wasn't any money left for getaway weekends, vacations, or other "extras." It seemed we were cornered in every area of our life.*

The diagnosis and treatment of infertility, as well as the pursuit of adoption, are expensive ventures. Testing, surgery, medication, in vitro fertilization (IVF) treatment, or living and medical costs for a birth mother can quickly consume thousands of dollars (see Table 3.1).

During their fertility treatment, most couples depend on their medical insurance to cover all or most of the expense. However, many insurance companies are now denying or curtailing coverage for infertility claims. For many, even partial responsibility for medical bills creates a financial hardship. To complicate matters, it's difficult to predict how much a medical procedure will cost. Each health provider or department, such as anesthesia, radiology, pharmacy, operating room, and surgeon,

TABLE 3.1 Costs of Infertility Tests, Treatments, and Adoption

Procedure	Charges*
Initial Visit, Interview, Physical Exam—Female	$125 plus any lab work ordered
Initial Visit, Interview, Physical Exam—Male	$85 plus any lab work ordered
Semen Analysis	$50–75
Post Coital Test (PCT)	$40–50 depending on length of office visit
Sperm Antibody Test	$100–150
Hysterosalpingogram	$185 for radiologist and hospital charges
Various Hormonal Blood Test for Women and Men	$46–60 depending on test
Testicular Biopsy	$240–300 or more for surgeon's fees plus anesthesiologist and hospital charges of $950
Endometrial Biopsy	$155 for physician's and laboratory charges
Hamster Egg Test (Sperm Penetration Assay)	$250
"Fertility Drug" Treatment with HMG (Pergonal)	$1000–1500 per cycle for drug and monitoring costs
Artificial Insemination by Donor (AID)	$150–200 per insemination
Laparoscopy	$2500 for surgeon, anesthesiologist and outpatient hospital charges
Gamete Intrafallopian Tube Transfer (GIFT)	About $3500 per attempt
In Vitro Fertilization (IVF)	Between $5000–8000 per attempt depending on procedures and individual program
Major Surgery for Removal of Tubal Blockages, Adhesions or Endometriosis	$3000 or more for surgeon, assistant surgeon, and anesthesiologist charges, plus hospital charges of $5,000 or more, depending on length of stay, time in operating room, medications, etc.
Vasectomy Reversal	$3000–5000 or more for surgeon, assistant surgeon, and anesthesiologist charges, plus hospital charges of $1000 or more, depending on whether done on outpatient basis, length of stay, etc.
Independent Adoption**	$5000 or more for living, counseling and medical costs for the birth mother and newborn, plus $2000 or more for attorney's fees and other legal costs.

TABLE 3.1 (continued)

Procedure	Charges*
Agency Adoption**	Varies from a few hundred dollars for some types of public agency adoptions to thousands of dollars for some private agency and international adoptions.
Surrogate Arrangements**	From about $11,000 for an arrangement based on the independent adoption model, to $25,000 or more when fees for surrogate and agency services are added.

* Costs vary in different locales. These charges based on an average of 1987 fees from several San Francisco area hospitals, physicians, and laboratories.
** Adoption and surrogate expenses based on an average of costs incurred in 1986 by several Northern California couples. Expenses vary in each situation.

usually submits separate bills, and may be impatient with queries about estimated costs. Furthermore it is difficult to predict the duration of surgery, how long the patient will stay in the hospital, or what supplies or drugs will be used. Couples pursuing open adoption face a similar dilemma. They cannot estimate the total cost of the birthmother or baby's living and medical expenses or even whether the placement will actually occur.

We are discovering that a certain level of affluence, combined with excellent medical insurance benefits, is necessary to challenge infertility. As costs escalate with inflation and advanced technology, increasing numbers of couples are being priced out of fertility treatment or adoption.

The denial of reimbursement for part or all of the treatment has culminated in an insurance crisis for infertile patients. For example, IVF (which often costs $5000 or more per attempt) is excluded from most policies. In addition many companies pay only a "usual and customary rate" (UCR) for medical fees. Because many specialists and hospitals charge in excess of the UCR, patients are billed directly for increasing percentages of their medical costs.

Consumer groups in a number of states are now rallying to fight the insurance crisis. They argue that covering infertility expenses would not significantly increase insurance industry costs. In fact infertility treatment and diagnosis account for only about $400,000,000 per year in the United States—less than 1 percent of total health care costs. (At present insurance carriers routinely cover such surgical family-planning procedures as sterilization and abortion.)

These groups organize concerned citizens at the grass roots level, obtain hundreds of letters of support, and educate and lobby legislators to draft bills that mandate coverage for infertility treatment. New York, Delaware, Massachusetts, and California are among the states that have either initiated or passed legislation requiring such coverage. Patient rights groups in other states are now organizing similar campaigns.

RESOLVE's national office is monitoring these efforts across the country. They can provide materials gathered from other states' efforts and network you with others concerned about this issue.

Low Income and Infertility

► *There is a widespread myth that only upper-middle-class, professional people have fertility problems. This is simply not true.*

Many low-income people who do not have medical insurance come to our clinic seeking fertility treatment. They desperately want to have a child but are without financial resources. I think this segment of the infertility population is largely ignored and forgotten.

MICHAEL POLICAR, M.D.
Medical Director, Planned Parenthood
of Alameda/San Francisco

Television and other media tend to portray the typical infertile couple as white, college-educated, and about 30 years old. Although a number of patients certainly fit this category, many low-income and working class people also suffer from fertility problems. Few have savings accounts or other sources of cash, and many are without medical insurance.

These patients also often encounter secondary infertility. Many have had one or more children in their teens or early twenties and then find themselves infertile later in life. Like other infertile women and men, they may also discover complications from previous miscarriages or abortions, tubal disease from sexually transmitted diseases, and endometriosis.

Federally Funded Infertility Services

In 1969 Congress passed the Public Health Service Act. Title X of this act provides funding for the Family Planning Services program. Under this program family planning clinics can apply for grants to provide patient education, contraception, and infertility counseling and diagnosis.

Initially funding was used to develop basic family planning programs, which focused primarily on contraception. Infertility counseling and education were added slowly as the government recognized the growing need for fertility services. At least one infertility program was funded in each of ten regions, and guidelines for infertility patient diagnosis and care were established:

- **Level 1:** A minimum infertility workup, which includes an interview, examination, appropriate lab work, patient education, counseling and appropriate referral
- **Level 2:** Semen analysis, assessment of ovulatory function (by BBT chart or endometrial biopsy), postcoital test
- **Level 3:** More sophisticated and complex testing and treatment

Unfortunately, total funding for the family planning programs has decreased with recent federal budget cuts. In 1986 the continuation level of funding allocated for all family planning programs (which include contraception, infertility diagnosis and patient counseling, education, and outreach) was $142.5 million. This amount was subject to a 4.3 percent Gramm-Rudman-Hollings cut later in the year. To compensate for this loss of revenue some clinics have reduced infertility services to the minimum Level 1 required by law; others have even curtailed this part of their program. Presently there is no available nationwide data of the services provided in each funded clinic.

There is, however, increasing sensitivity among many federal administrators about our nation's growing infertility problem. Patients who qualify can still locate clinics that offer basic testing and counseling on a sliding scale or no-fee basis. In addition sympathetic physicians and hospitals often volunteer time for these programs and may offer long-term payment plans to patients who require surgery or medications.

State Assistance

Some states provide funding for infertility services to those who qualify as low-income patients; unfortunately many of these programs exclude single women. Patients may be eligible for infertility testing (up to but usually not including laparoscopy) and some medications such as clomiphene or HMG. Funds may also be available to train nurse practitioners in basic infertility testing under the supervision of a physician.

Locating a Federal or State Infertility Program

Contact the nearest federal regional office of family planning services for information about infertility services in your area (see Appendix B).

Because some states also earmark funds for infertility testing and diagnosis, call your state's department of health or family planning services for information. You can usually find their number in your phone book under Department of Health in the section containing state offices.

Also check the yellow pages for family planning programs and prenatal clinics, which may provide referrals to infertility programs, physicians, and hospitals that provide care on a sliding scale according to ability to pay.

The Right to Infertility Treatment for All

Information, emotional support, and competent medical care should be available to all patients who experience fertility problems. Beverly Freeman, executive director of RESOLVE, Inc., urges those who have encountered infertility in a personal or professional way to help in this effort.

In addition to legislation mandating insurance coverage for infertility, employers can be encouraged to subsidize medical and adoption costs. Federal and state legislators must also be educated about the needs of all patients and urged to work for increased funding for low-income infertility clinics.

CHAPTER 4

The Doctor-Patient Relationship

► *I have the greatest confidence in my doctor. Without his knowledge and kindness, I would not have felt this way. I went into surgery knowing that if anyone could help me, he could.*

► *Our meeting with the doctor about artificial insemination by donor was very impersonal. A lot of notes were made about my husband's physical characteristics, the procedure itself was discussed, and we were asked when we wanted to start. Just like that! I asked if there was counseling available to sort through our feelings. He actually laughed and said couples had no business in his clinic if they had doubts. He wasn't allowing at all for any normal apprehensions.*

► *Many people say to me, "You must be so happy when your infertility patients get pregnant!" Sure, I share their excitement, but my heart is really with those patients who try all the treatments and don't get pregnant.*

As these quotes suggest, the doctor-patient relationship is often a personal and sensitive one. We look to our physicians for competent medical care, understanding, and compassion, and we hope they will come to know us. Some patients return to the same internist or family practitioner for many years, and close bonds often develop between them.

Because physicians are highly educated, have prominent social status, and often appear harried or rushed, many patients are also intimidated or awed by them. We may feel nervous, tongue-tied, or uncomfortable in their presence. Some of us find it difficult to ask questions, express concerns, or discuss a suggested treatment during office visits or phone conversations.

Infertility patients approach their specialists with these feelings, as well as with hope and apprehension. Each couple wants to have a child and depends on the doctor to help them achieve this life goal. Although they worry that testing or perhaps surgery will be necessary, they also fear that pregnancy won't occur even after these procedures. Patients who have unsuccessfully seen other physicians often bring a demoralized attitude to the initial interview. The specialist senses their expectations and unhappiness and is frustrated when patients do not respond to treatment.

It is easy to see how resentments, misunderstandings, conflicts, and hurt feelings can surface on both sides. From the outset, the doctor-patient relationship is loaded with high physical, emotional, psychological, and financial stakes.

Underlying this relationship is a challenge that we infertility patients take responsibility for our own health care. This approach requires careful selection of a competent specialist and continuous self-education about our medical problems and proposed treatments. In addition, a commitment from both physician and patient to open communication, realistic expectations, sensitivity to the other's perspective, and an attitude of mutual respect and trust can strengthen the doctor-patient relationship.

Choosing an Infertility Specialist

► *We wasted months with our gynecologist. He wanted to stick with BBT charts, clomiphene, and simple tests. At no time did he suggest a laparoscopy.*

We'd finally had enough and decided to see an infertility specialist. We had to wait quite awhile for an appointment, but it was worth it. We've often joked that it was like the difference between a Vega and a Bentley. Our specialist was thorough and concerned. He gave us hope without being condescending or glib. After he found massive pelvic adhesions caused by chronic appendicitis, he recommended surgery to increase our chances for pregnancy. At last we had a diagnosis and something to do about it.

All licensed physicians have completed four years of medical school and passed board-approved examinations. After a year of internship, some choose a specialty such as obstetrics and gynecology (ob/gyn). Specializing in a specific area of medicine requires a three- to four-year residency to obtain additional knowledge and clinical experience.

Although infertility has been a recognized subspecialty of gynecology since 1974, not all ob/gyns are adequately educated or trained in infertility diagnosis and treatment. Many medical students receive only one course or perhaps several relevant lectures while in medical school and little surgical or clinical infertility training during their residency.

What Is an Infertility Specialist?

Infertility specialists are physicians who have received additional education, training, and experience in the diagnosis and treatment of infertility beyond the ob/gyn residency. Some have completed a two-year clinical fellowship in Reproductive Endocrinology. Others acquire knowledge and training through seminars and other continuing medical education. They devote all or part of their practice to fertility problems, keep abreast of current technological developments in the field, and perform infertility surgery and complex testing on a regular basis. These specialists are best qualified to diagnose and treat all aspects of female and male infertility, except for male fertility surgery, which is referred to a urologist.

When Should I See a Specialist?

Many couples regret wasting months or even years of precious time with well-intentioned internists or gynecologists who were not qualified to diagnose or treat infertility.

You should consider a consultation with an infertility specialist if:

- You have not become pregnant after a year of unprotected intercourse.
- You have suffered three or more miscarriages.
- Your infertility is affecting your marital relationship or either partner's self-esteem.

How Do I Find a Specialist?

Your gynecologist or internist may be able to refer you to an infertility specialist in your area. In addition, RESOLVE has compiled a *Directory of Infertility Resources,* an updated listing of specialists across the country. Many local chapters can also provide referrals. RESOLVE recommends that an infertility specialist should have at least half of his or her practice devoted to infertility.

What Are the Qualities of a Good Specialist?

You may want to interview several specialists before selecting one. This is a sensitive relationship in which you will discuss personal aspects of your health, feelings, and sexuality and make important decisions about testing, treatment, and perhaps surgery.

We all want a competent doctor who is experienced in infertility diagnosis and treatment and trained in the current medical technology. Your specialist should also be aware of the powerful emotional and psychological dynamics of infertility that can affect the doctor-patient relationship. Misunderstandings can be minimized or avoided through continuing dialogue with a sensitive specialist.

Other important qualities to look for during your first few contacts include:

- A willingness and availability to answer your questions during office visits and by telephone (as time allows).
- Arrangements with other infertility specialists to cover for vacations, days off, evenings, or weekends.
- A professional and personal rapport with you as a patient and with you both as a couple.
- The desire to work with both of you on the course of the workup and possible treatments.
- A friendly, sensitive staff with whom you feel comfortable discussing your concerns.
- An honest discussion of fees before testing or surgery and an arrangement for payment that is acceptable to all.
- An efficiently run office where you are seen within a reasonable time of your scheduled appointment.

Educating Yourself about Infertility

► *I think all infertility patients should be thoroughly acquainted with their problem and its management. This requires learning as much as possible through reading and discussion. Good infertility specialists know they must take appropriate time to talk with their patients. However, we doctors are frequently hurried and it may sometimes be necessary for the patient to initiate questions.*

Learning about the medical, as well as the emotional, issues of your infertility often restores a sense of control. This knowledge can ease fears about proposed tests or surgery and provide reassurance about the intensity of your feelings. Your reading, however, will not make you a medical expert. Your specialist has spent years studying these problems and their treatment; the purpose of your research is not to outsmart or second-guess the specialist, but to give you a base of knowledge that, along with your doctor's recommendations, can help you make informed decisions.

A word of warning is necessary however. Reading about health problems, particularly in medical journals, can be unnerving or frightening. In fact medical students often suffer from sympathetic hypochrondria when they study certain problems! As a lay reader you may also interpret medical data incorrectly. For example, some articles report the results of only one study rather than a comprehensive overview. If you are confused or alarmed by what you've read, discuss your concerns with your doctor.

Getting Started

Ask your specialist for recommendations of relevant books and journal articles, and check local bookstores for their latest titles on infertility. The public library also offers a wealth of resources. Consult the card catalog, video display screens, and the *Reader's Guide to Periodical Literature* (under the subject heading Infertility or specific medical complaints, such as Pelvic Inflammatory Disease) for books and magazine articles for the lay reader. Each reference will probably recommend other readings on the same subject.

Fact sheets on specific medical problems are available from RESOLVE. There are also several medical research services, that for a fee, will send you detailed information on a specific topic. One of these is Planetree Health Resource Center, which also has a medical library and bookstore (see Appendix A). Your doctor, pharmacist, nurses, and other health care providers may also be helpful.

Using the Medical Library

You can find more specialized, technical books and journal articles—written by and for physicians and other health care professionals—in a medical library. These libraries are found in some universities and most nursing and medical schools and are usually open to the public.

The card catalog lists books by author, title, and subject. Articles specific to your interest can be found by using *Index Medicus,* an annually compiled index that lists articles published in all national and some international medical journals by author, subject, and title. Recent journal issues are usually shelved alphabetically by journal title. Older editions are bound, stored in the stacks, and also filed alphabetically by journal title. If you need help, ask the reference librarian.

You can read about specific drugs in the *Physicians' Desk Reference* (PDR) and the *Medical Letter.* The PDR is an annual publication that compiles information from the manufacturers about indications for, and all reported side effects of, various drugs. Designed for use by physicians, the PDR contains a lot of medical jargon, lists hundreds of rare side effects as well as common ones, and may be difficult or even disturbing reading. The *Medical Letter* is a periodical that evaluates various drugs on the market and also lists references to appropriate journal articles and other readings. The *Hospital Formulary* and *Essential Guide to Prescription Drugs* are other sources of information about prescription drugs. Each is written for pharmacists and physicians and may be difficult for the average reader to understand.

Infertility Patient's Perspective

► *I remember the first time I saw the sign on the door: "Joe Jones, M.D., Obstetrics, Gynecology, Infertility." I felt a sinking feeling because I hated admitting I was infertile and that I needed medical help to get pregnant.*

I wanted to get out of that role as soon as possible and become an ob patient. But my infertility dragged on even though we progressed quickly through the workup and major surgery.

I kept at it, though, going monthly for postcoital tests and pelvic exams while I took clomiphene. I soon associated my frequent office visits with failure, inadequacy, and depression.

My doctor's moods also varied with each visit. Sometimes I sensed that he was optimistic about my chances; other times I felt he was also depressed and didn't really know what to say to me.

I remember one occasion when he called me and reported a positive test result. I sensed that he was relieved, and for once, I felt hope because something was normal. I said to him, "Now do you think I'll get pregnant?"

His attitude changed immediately. He became very serious and said, "We make no guarantees here about pregnancy. It's very important for you understand that."

My elation disappeared and I again felt infertile.

All transitions can be unsettling and even frightening. Infertility is an especially unhappy and difficult one. During this "time window" of our lives, we are struggling with the reality that we cannot easily conceive or birth a child. It is a sad time and one we wish to end quickly. Regardless of our commitment or diligence, however, there is no guarantee of a pregnancy.

By the time most patients see a specialist they are already frightened, anxious, and perhaps desperate. Some are ashamed to be seeing a specialist at all. Many fear they'll never get pregnant, whether they've been trying for several months or years. They are all reacting to a myriad of stresses and may not have found adequate emotional support. On top of all this few begin the workup with much medical knowledge. In fact this may be their first experience with a physical problem that requires treatment.

Attitude Toward the Specialist

Every infertility patient hopes this will be a short-term relationship. We want the specialist to restore our fertility so we can become pregnant. As the workup and treatment progress, this perspective can result in several differing attitudes toward the physician.

Some patients are awed by doctors and view them as all-knowing miracle workers. They often expect the doctor to take total responsibility for their health care and fear giving offense by complaining, airing their feelings, or being "a nuisance." Some patients are afraid that if they are too pushy, their specialist won't see them anymore. AID (artificial insemination by donor) patients often feel especially dependent on the doctor. Their specialist may be the only person aware of their insemination treatments and often selects the donor who will be their child's biological father.

Other patients look toward their specialist for emotional support. Because the doctor must maintain a certain amount of professional and personal distance, such patients are often disappointed. Some patients complain that their specialists are cold or unfeeling about their emotional pain and feel frustrated or let down after office visits or phone conversations.

Still other patients take a cold, rather callous view of their physicians. They may resent the specialist's emotional detachment, high fees, bedside manner, or fertility symbolized by the pictures of his or her children in the office. Some treat physicians like professional athletes, showing interest only in the specialist's record of pregnancy successes. This may be their one chance for a child and they fear selecting a physician with a low success rate.

In any case every infertility patient wants and perhaps expects a miracle: a pregnancy despite medical problems, prognosis, or age. Many become disillusioned, impatient, and angry if this doesn't occur within a few months of treatment. The fact that it may take several years for a successful pregnancy to occur (if at all) can be hard to accept. As time passes, it is a challenge to maintain a positive attitude toward both the specialist and the course of treatment.

Physician's Perspective

► *It's often discouraging for me to practice this form of medicine. I know my patients want only one thing from me: fertility. But I also know the numbers: Less than half of them will have a successful pregnancy.*

This is hard to accept for all of us. The joy of working with these couples is that they're the best patients in the world and follow your instructions to the letter. If I tell my patients that the latest infertility cure is to stand on your head on the sidewalk at high noon, they'll only ask, "Should I put a towel on the ground or just place my forehead directly on the cement?"

It's heartbreaking for me when they don't succeed.

Infertility specialists are responsible for the care and treatment of many patients. They often work closely, for months at a time, with the patient or couple. As a rule these model patients are diligent, dependable, and cooperative. They usually keep their appointments; follow instructions exactly; undergo necessary tests; take their medications as ordered; and, if asked, chart their daily basal temperature for months or years on end! Specialists develop an emotional attachment to many of their patients.

Emotionally infertility is one of the more difficult medical specialties to practice. It is a heartbreaking reality that only about half these patients will become pregnant. In fact many specialists actually have a lower success rate—perhaps 30 to 40 percent. This is because the more fertile patients often become pregnant while under the care of their gynecologists. The cases referred to a specialist are usually more difficult and have smaller chances for success. The physician may keenly feel the couple's successes and failures, along with their disappointment when fertility remains an elusive goal. In fact it can be difficult for both physician and patient to decide whether to try yet another option or end treatment.

Despite their commitment and sympathy, however, physicians must maintain a professional distance from each patient. Otherwise it would be impossible to see a dozen or more new and returning patients each day, perform surgery several times a week, and meet the demands and needs of their own families.

Bedside Manner

Each physician develops his or her own bedside manner—a personalized way of conveying expertise, reassurance, and sympathy to patients. Some doctors use a frank and honest approach both in explaining medical problems and in expressing their own feelings. Others are more reserved, preferring a more formal doctor-patient relationship with little show of emotion. Patients' reactions to their physicians also differ widely. Some like a gentle, reassuring manner; others prefer to hear the straight facts and skip any show of emotion.

Many doctors are cautious about expressing feelings or confidences, aware that patients often discuss physicians and their personalities with friends and acquaintances. It's also difficult to judge how much encouragement or hope to hold out to a patient. Even among patients with a favorable prognosis, many do not become pregnant.

Nurses and Other Health Care Professionals

► *Suspecting an ectopic pregnancy, I made an appointment with a gyn colleague whose work I highly respect. The unhurried, sincere concern I sensed from the physician, as well as the thoroughness of his examinations, were immensely reassuring. I reproached myself, as a nurse, for every time I had depersonalized patients in dealing with their concerns, often edging out the door as I answered their questions.*

► *Few patients realize how many demands are placed on the nursing staff. One nurse will often have three or four patients who need attention, help, or medications at the same time. Our patients also tend to express their anger and resentment about the hospital, their illness, or life in general to us, rather than their doctors. I try my best to be cheerful, efficient, and reassuring to my patients. But I can only be in one place at a time, and I have good and bad days like everybody else.*

It hurts when patients are rude or critical, although I know that being hospitalized is traumatic and unsettling. I also wonder what happens to patients after they are discharged. Few call back or write to let me know how they're doing. When someone does, it means a lot.

During infertility testing and treatment patients see a number of health care providers such as nurses, lab technicians, and medical assistants. Although these are short-term relationships, they can influence your medical experience.

Through the course of a day or night these providers are responsible for the care of many people. They realize that patients, either in the doctor's office or a hospital setting, are often tense and unhappy. Still it is painful when patients treat them in an insensitive manner or consider their work and feelings unimportant. They may also be frustrated by their brief contact with patients. Unlike the physician they don't know how patients fare after testing or surgery.

Some patients are not aware of the many demands on the care provider's time and emotions. Often a nurse's hurried manner or tense body language is misinterpreted as a lack of concern toward the patient. It is comforting when nurses take the time to explain a medical procedure or offer reassurance and a kind word.

There are times when nurses or technicians *are* insensitive or unkind, or patients are unnecessarily rude or short-tempered. When problems occur, either party should try an honest statement of feelings and expectations. If this doesn't work, a patient might discuss the problem with her or his physician. Nurses can air their feelings with their supervisors and physicians.

Building a Relationship of Mutual Respect and Trust

► *It is only through the development of an honest, respectful, and informed relationship that the needs of infertility patients can be met. I think most of my colleagues are aware of this and appreciate active patient participation. It is also important to realize that sometimes specific answers are not available, and both doctor and patient must live with less-than-optimal information. Even in these cases your doctor should be able to put the clinical situation into perspective so you can make appropriate decisions regarding management of your infertility problem.*

► *For months I thought I was just another patient to my specialist. During my treatment I've gone through many emotions over dozens of visits: anger, hope, frustration, fear, depression, gratitude. At first I figured he really didn't care how depressed I was, how I often left his office and cried for hours. After I told him how I felt (months later), he admitted that he too was sad and depressed by my continuing fertility problems but didn't know how to express that.*

We both changed over time, after lots of conversations. I came to expect less, he to give more. All told he has spent long hours talking to me and, in surgery, trying to heal my body. After my surgery, he was at the hospital day and night, monitoring my progress. He even had the lab call him at home during the night with my blood test results. He tried everything medically possible to enable me to get pregnant. And finally he offered me emotional support.

I'll never forget all he did for me. I wish I knew the words to tell him of my gratitude and how very, very special he is.

Given the different perspectives of specialist and patient, and the highly charged issues of infertility, it is not surprising that misunderstandings can and do arise. There aren't any pat answers or suggestions for the ideal doctor-patient relationship. Depending on the length and intensity of your treatment and the personalities involved, stressful and unhappy moments can occur in even the best situation. The following suggestions are offered as a base for building a partnership of mutual respect and trust that can withstand the inevitable stresses of infertility.

Clear Objectives and Teamwork

Optimally the couple and specialist clarify the goals for diagnosis and treatment early in the workup. After some education about the suspected problem, the couple must decide which treatments are acceptable. If they cannot agree on how much or how long to investigate their infertility, a consultation with a qualified therapist may be helpful.

The couple should keep their specialist apprised of their wishes and objectives. After the workup is completed, the physician will make recommendations for treatment. Working together they can weigh the chances of success, expense, and risk of each suggested procedure and plan an appropriate course of action.

Honest, Open Communication

Patients often complain that their physicians don't take the time to answer their questions or explain medical problems adequately. Even after several conversations some patients don't fully understand their medical problem or why a certain treatment has been recommended. Others are distressed when the doctor doesn't return their calls within a few hours. This can be especially frustrating if a patient is waiting for a test result or has a specific worry.

On the other hand, physicians often observe that some patients don't ask questions or voice their concerns during office visits but want to spend an hour or so on the phone later that day. Doctors also feel that many patients take out their frustration with infertility on them and ignore their competent medical care.

Both specialist and patient should feel comfortable in stating expectations and concerns as they arise. Because it is easy to forget details when you are nervous or sense the doctor is rushed, it may be helpful to write down questions before office visits. Ask your physician to simplify any medical language you don't understand. Attend visits with your mate whenever possible. Your partner often catches information or suggestions that you have missed and may remember questions you meant to ask.

If a misunderstanding occurs, try to discuss the situation as soon as possible. An honest exchange of feelings, with sensitivity to each other's perspective, often results in a workable compromise. However, personality clashes do occur. A patient may be put off by a physician's impersonal bedside manner. The specialist, on the other hand, may sense resentment or hostility in the patient's attitude. Sometimes each party can bend a little and change his or her approach. This would certainly be the most desirable outcome, particularly if both doctor and patient have invested a lot of time, testing, and money in the relationship. If a compromise can't be reached, it may be best to see another specialist. In that case, be sure to obtain a copy of your medical records, including test and surgery reports.

Realistic Expectations on Both Sides

Infertility patients often enter this relationship with unrealistic expectations. Many assume that the specialist will:

- Immediately determine the cause of their infertility and fix the problem expertly and quickly.
- Be cheerful, supportive, and optimistic during each office visit and phone conversation.
- Be available at their convenience for discussions or procedures.

Many also expect a pregnancy a month or two after beginning treatment. When any or all of these hopes are not realized, patients often feel disappointed, misled, or angry.

Most specialists find it difficult to meet their patients', as well as their own, high expectations. They must also balance each patient's demands for information, reassurance, and emotional support against the needs and impatience of those sitting in the waiting room. Every specialist sees a wide spectrum of fertility problems among his or her patients. Some have a fairly good chance for pregnancy, while others are faced with a poor prognosis. Yet each patient probably feels 100 percent infertile, depressed, and emotionally vulnerable.

Infertility patients, often in emotional pain, sometimes become self-centered, panicky, and extremely demanding of the specialist's time and energy. Some expect their physicians to be available at all hours for questions or treatment and a few even request a copy of his or her schedule for months ahead! Many physicians feel guilty about taking vacations or time off, fearing that they won't "be there" for their patients. Others fear they will be unfairly blamed when treatment is unsuccessful.

Physicians can also hold unrealistic expectations. Many expect their patients to:

- Listen stoically to a poor prognosis.
- Suppress their physical and emotional pain even during stressful tests or surgeries.
- Organize their thoughts and ask intelligent questions regardless of their state of mind.
- Expect no emotional support.
- Follow their expert advice without question.

To build a positive relationship both doctor and patient should strive toward reasonable goals. The patient should expect the specialist to perform a competent and timely workup and provide expert advice on appropriate treatments, risks, costs, and success rates. Lengthy waits should be minimized, and when an emergency occurs, an appointment should be rescheduled as soon as possible. The specialist should reasonably expect that patients will take responsibility for health care and self-education (to some degree) about the problem and proposed treatments, initiate discussion, and speak up when concerned or confused.

Ideally, over the course of this relationship both doctor and patient learn to respect each other's strengths and limitations. Both can recognize that there is no guarantee of a pregnancy, and although the specialist can provide medical expertise and some emotional support, the couple alone must undergo the treatments and resolve their situation. Whatever warmth, caring, and encouragement the specialist can bring to the relationship helps the couple face their reality.

Whether or not a pregnancy occurs, they have both done their very best.

CHAPTER 5

Surgery

► *I've been to surgery five times. With each experience, I've learned a lot about myself and those around me. Each time I thought, "I can't possibly go through with this," but I did. And each time those in my life gave me their love, flowers, poems, and homemade soup to heal me.*

I don't think I've ever felt such absolute terror as while I waited outside the operating room. I know I've never felt such happiness and relief as when I awoke from the anesthesia, and thought, "It's so good to be alive."

I've felt hatred and disgust with my body because fertility surgery was necessary. I've also felt pride and love for the strength of my legs and the force of my will as I got up from the bed and took those first painful, shuffling, independent steps.

I think surgery is the ultimate physical, emotional, and spiritual experience, perhaps like going into combat. You are depending on your body to survive, counting on your heart and mind to hold you together, and trusting in God that it will all be worthwhile.

Many infertility patients require some type of surgery. Laparoscopy, for example, is a diagnostic tool of the female infertility workup and a standard procedure for in vitro fertilization. Many women undergo surgery for adhesion removal, tubal repair, endometriosis, fibroid tumors, and ovarian cysts. Most fertility surgery is performed on women, although some men also undergo surgery for testicular biopsy, varicocele, or vasectomy reversal.

Infertility patients may require either minor or major surgery. Minor surgery, often performed in an hour or two under appropriate anesthesia, is usually done on an outpatient basis. This means you are admitted and released from the hospital on the same day. Most patients recover fairly quickly, and physical activities may be limited for only a few days. (See Chapter 8 for a discussion of laparoscopy as outpatient surgery.)

Major fertility surgery, on the other hand, usually involves an abdominal incision, an operation of several hours or longer performed under general anesthesia, and inpatient hospitalization of four or more days. Physical activity is limited for up to six weeks afterward.

Although this chapter has been written largely from the female perspective, the reactions and feelings surgery evokes are universal to all patients. It is a traumatic event in a physical, emotional, and psychological sense. Because the body will be cut open, it is a frightening, invasive experience. Nearly all of us regard an upcoming operation with apprehension and dread. We realize this is a risk; serious complications can result from even minor surgery or local anesthesia. Infertility surgery also raises unique hopes and fears. In most cases our lives or health are not threatened, yet we risk elective surgery in hopes of increasing our chances for pregnancy. At the same time surgery on our reproductive organs elicits an almost primal, visceral reaction that closely touches our sexual identities and self-images. This surgery may be critical to our future ability to reproduce, and many of us pin our hopes and dreams of producing a biological child on the success of the attempt. Although the long-term emotional, physical, and financial costs are high, nearly all of us fantasize that this effort will lead to a pregnancy.

Deciding on Major Surgery

► *The idea of having major surgery frightened me. I was afraid to have my body cut open and to stay in the hospital. But my laparoscopy showed extensive adhesions and my chances for pregnancy were very small. I wanted to give myself the best chance and was excited by the thought that this would lead to a pregnancy. After a lot of soul searching, I decided to try the surgery.*

The decision to undergo major surgery is a difficult one. It is a significant commitment in terms of time, disability, emotional stress, and money. Even if the surgery is covered by medical insurance, infertility patients are often responsible for portions of their surgeon's and hospital bills.

In most cases infertility surgery will be elective. It is not necessary to maintain your health but may improve your chances for pregnancy. In other situations, such as ectopic pregnancy, malignancy, or large tumors or cysts, major surgery may be necessary to prevent serious complications.

In any event selecting a competent and emotionally supportive infertility specialist is of the utmost importance (see Chapter 4). Once a specific problem has been identified, you and your mate can work closely with the specialist to weigh the advantages and drawbacks of available treatments. You may also want a second opinion from another competent infertility specialist. Most physicians will respect your decision to obtain another opinion before consenting to surgery.

You may also want to speak with other patients who have had this type of surgery. Your specialist or local RESOLVE chapter can usually refer you to others willing to discuss their surgical experiences. They can provide the patient's perspective on the physical, emotional, and psychological aspects of the type of surgery you are considering.

Ultimately this is your decision, though it will elicit lots of discussion, suggestions, and advice from family and friends. Once your decision is made, trust your instincts and politely but firmly table any further discussion.

Preoperative Hopes and Fears

► *I daydreamed about a successful outcome. I saw myself walking in the sunshine with a big, very pregnant belly. It would all be worthwhile.*

► *I feared the surgery. The idea of my reproductive organs being operated on was terrifying. I was also confused and angry that my body was ill. I had a hard time sleeping at night and often lay awake thinking and worrying. What if something went wrong? I'd never get pregnant.*

Most of us approach infertility surgery with hope, faith, and excitement and fantasize about being one of the lucky successes. It's natural to feel positive and hopeful as one prepares for surgery. It would be hard to go through with it without that boost. Still it is sensible to be realistic. As you prepare for surgery, investigate and discuss other infertility resolutions as contingency plans.

Surgical patients generally feel apprehensive as the date of their scheduled operation approaches; a number of powerful emotions may surface and patients often:

- Feel confused, angry, or frightened because their bodies are ill and surgery is required. They wonder, "Why me? What did I do to deserve this?"

- Fear that their fertility and, perhaps, sexuality are at stake. Compounding this fear is the knowledge that surgery is a gamble. Many patients remark that if they only *knew* this effort would result in a pregnancy, they would not hesitate to try. The reality is that there is no guarantee of a successful pregnancy.
- Fear that something will go wrong during the anesthesia or surgery and result in complications or even death.
- Worry they will not "behave properly" during the hospital stay, that they'll cry, lose control, or reveal embarrassing secrets while semiconscious.
- Worry about the effect of the surgery on their marriages and whether their mates will be understanding and helpful during the hospital stay and convalescence.

Many patients experience preop anxiety symptoms such as crying, sleeping disorders, irritability, obsession with the decision, or free-floating anxiety. It helps to:

- Make a list of your worries. Keep paper and pencil handy around the house, in your purse or pocket, and near your bed. Jot down thoughts as they occur to you. Fears often surface during late night and early morning hours when you try to sleep. Don't fight your insomnia. Switch on the light, write down your worries as they come to mind, and then reorder them by magnitude, with number one being your greatest fear. Let the paper hold your worries until morning.
- Take positive, assertive steps to alleviate some of these fears. Start by reviewing your list with your specialist, who may be able to provide reassuring answers, emotional support, and perhaps referrals to hospital staff who can answer your questions about policy and routine.
- Speak with someone who has had surgery at your hospital. Former patients can apprise you of current hospital routine and quality of care.
- Prepare your body and mind for the surgery. Chapter 7 discusses the importance of physical and emotional fitness when coping with infertility. This is doubly important before surgery. Regular exercise, proper nutrition, and relaxation exercises build strength and stamina, release tension, and optimize your chances for a successful surgery and speedy convalescence.
- A day or two before surgery, you will have a preop appointment with your specialist to ensure that you are in good physical health and with-

out any medical problems that may affect the surgery. This appointment is also a good time to discuss your concerns. If you have further questions afterward, call your doctor.

The Hospital Experience

► *The medical care before and after my surgery was wonderful. The nurses were friendly, concerned, and empathetic. My specialist and anesthesiologist visited me the evening before surgery to answer my questions and reassure me. After the operation the nurses encouraged me to get out of bed, showed me how to manage the IV stand, and walked along with me down the hall. They helped me shower and wash my hair, respected my dignity, and treated me in a sensitive manner. When I was discharged, they came in to say goodbye and predicted my next stay would be in maternity. They asked me to bring my baby to their floor to visit. I left feeling hopeful and well taken care of.*

► *I was taken downstairs to surgery on a wheeled stretcher and left in the waiting area with several semiconscious patients. I felt alone and frightened. I noticed a group of orderlies and nurses standing a few feet away, laughing and talking. I wished someone would say something comforting to me, but they didn't seem to notice me, and I was too embarrassed to speak to them first. I heard them discuss an unpleasant abortion performed the day before. I was angered by their insensitivity and the hospital's policy, which left patients lying alone as they waited their turn for surgery.*

I later wrote a letter of complaint to the chairman of the hospital's board of directors. A few weeks later I received courteous replies from both the chairman and the head surgical nurse. They both apologized for my experience and said they would speak to the surgical staff about their behavior. They were also considering policy changes that would allow support people in the surgery waiting area.

As these two stories illustrate, patients' hospital experiences can and do differ. Your feelings about your stay will be influenced by your attitude upon admission, the hospital's philosophy and policy, the number of staff on duty, and their competency and demeanor.

Some patients are familiar with hospitals and have positive feelings about them. They may have had favorable experiences in the past or may work in the health care field. Others regard hospitals as antiseptic, depersonalized, and depressing institutions and associate them with sickness or even death. Even under the best of circumstances major surgery is a difficult, confining experience. Previous fears or unpleasant memories of hospitals can result in greater preop apprehension.

In the past decade many hospitals have made significant changes in philosophy. They now permit the involvement of loved ones in the surgical experience and have extended visiting hours. Before surgery you may want to visit your hospital to become acquainted with its current policies.

Preregistration Forms

Most hospitals mail a preregistration packet a few weeks before your scheduled surgery. The enclosed forms ask about insurance coverage, room preference, and relevant health concerns for the anesthesiologist and nursing staff.

WHAT TYPE OF ROOM? You can usually request a private or semiprivate (two beds) room or a ward (three or more beds) for your stay. There are both benefits and drawbacks to all three options.

A private room affords solitude and privacy, which many of us prefer when our strength and emotions are low. In a private room we avoid a roommate's visitors, complaints, and phone, television, and personal habits. Many hospitals allow a spouse or friend to "room-in" and will provide a cot for overnight stays. Some patients work out a schedule in advance with friends and relatives for each day of their hospital stay to provide assistance, emotional support, and companionship.

There are, however, several disadvantages to a private room. It can be lonely. If your mate or family should leave for a few hours or overnight, you are on your own. This can be particularly isolating the first few days after surgery when you are most dependent on others. Some hospitals have also reduced the number of nurses on each shift, so those on duty are often overworked and unable to give patients much attention.

Most medical insurance policies cover only the cost of a semiprivate room and require that you make up the difference for a private one, usually an additional $30 or $40 per day. The hospital may have only a few private rooms, and one may not be available the day you are admitted.

A semiprivate room or ward provides companionship. If you are on a floor for postsurgical care, you may find empathetic roommates with similar histories and experiences. Short- or even long-term friendships can develop. On the other hand you may not be compatible with your roommate. Four days or longer in a difficult rooming situation can seem like an eternity, but you can request a room change if necessary.

Interacting with Hospital Staff

During your hospital stay you will interact with nurses, surgical teams, lab technicians, volunteers, and other hospital staff. How they treat you, both medically and emotionally, affects your experience.

The number of nurses on duty after surgery and the various crises they must cope with will also affect the quality of your postop stay. Many nurses are dedicated professionals, frustrated by the economic cutbacks that result in staffing shortages. At times they must prioritize patients according to the urgency of their needs and cannot always give each the care and attention both nurses and patients would like. Unless it is an emergency, some patients may need to wait before a nurse is able to answer their page or check their progress. If you should experience poor or substandard care, contact the nursing supervisor while you are in the hospital and mention your concerns to your specialist. Sometimes the problem can be worked out at the time.

Suggestions for Your Hospital Stay

Thoughtful and careful advance planning can ease the stress of a hospital stay. The following suggestions are offered by patients who have had major surgery:

- Pack your suitcase a few days in advance. You'll need several nightgowns or pajama sets; underwear; socks, legwarmers; a bathrobe; slippers; and jogging pants, caftans, or other loose-fitting clothes. Do not bring jewelry, money, stereo equipment, TVs, or other valuables. Unfortunately theft is as much a problem in hospitals as it is in the rest of the world.
- Add warmth and color to your room by packing some happy reminders of home, such as photographs of loved ones, favorite books, or a familiar afghan or blanket.
- Bring stationery, notecards, and your journal. Surgery is usually a powerful experience, and you may want to write to friends or jot some thoughts down. If you don't have a journal, consider keeping one for this experience. Ask the nurses to insert your IV needle on your non-writing hand or wrist. Also pack a few books or magazines.
- Bring your address and telephone book. Most hospitals provide a telephone by each bed, and you can usually make as many local calls as you wish. Long distance or toll calls can be charged either to your home phone or credit calling card.
- Many hospital dieticians offer a wide variety of nutritious, appetizing foods for postoperative diets. Others offer only an adequate selection

of "institutional" food. After surgery you will be offered a sample of various menus according to your physician's instructions. Once you are back on a regular diet, you'll want to assess this fare for fresh vegetables, fruits, and whole grains. With your physician's approval, consider enriching the hospital diet with food and vitamin supplements.

Inpatient Surgery

► *I felt like a little girl again going to have my tonsils out—a little afraid and a little happy because the doctor would make me all better. The surgery prep nurse shaved me from under my breasts down to my thighs. All my pubic hair was gone. Little by little my pride was going too. I started to feel that my control of the situation was quickly fading.*

Inpatient surgery involves a stay of one or more nights in the hospital and is usually scheduled several weeks in advance. When a diagnostic laparoscopy has been performed prior to this procedure, many specialists prefer to schedule major surgery four to six weeks later. Major surgery, which involves an abdominal incision of several inches (laparotomy), usually requires four or more days of inpatient recovery. Surgical treatment for endometriosis, tubal repair, varicocele, adhesion removal, ectopic pregnancy, and fibroid tumors commonly requires several hours or more of major surgery.

Checking Into the Hospital

Many patients are admitted to the hospital the afternoon or evening before, or the morning of, their scheduled surgery. In either case the admissions office is usually the first stop. Your preop questionnaire will be reviewed, medical insurance coverage confirmed and money due for private rooms or noncovered services collected. Your luggage will be tagged with your name and room number. You can also check valuables into the hospital safe, although it's best to leave them home.

A hospital volunteer may accompany you to either the laboratory or your hospital room. Blood work and other lab tests may be performed now, although many hospitals schedule preliminary lab work a few days before admission.

When you reach your floor, a nurse will greet you and show you to your room. Most hospital rooms have a closet, set of drawers, television, and phone for each patient, as well as a bathroom with toilet, sink, and shower for the occupants to share. Dinner is served in the early evening, and you can usually order a tray for a guest if you let a nurse know well in advance. You will also be asked to sign consent forms that list in detail the possible complications of anesthesia and surgery. Although the odds of such occurrences are small, these forms are frightening to read. Discuss any concerns with your specialist or anesthesiologist. They will both visit early this evening to discuss the surgery, answer questions, and reassure you. Most specialists offer their patients a sedative or sleeping pill to help them relax the evening before surgery.

Preparations for Surgery

Before pelvic surgery, most patients are shaved from the navel to the pubic area to ensure a sterile surgical area. Your vagina or penis will look different and strange without the surrounding pubic hair, but it grows back quickly.

Most surgeons also prescribe an enema to clear the bowels. This helps prevent abdominal cramping or complications during and after surgery. The nurses are experienced with this unpleasant, but relatively painless procedure, and are sensitive to your embarrassment. After the enema is finished, you can shower and prepare for bed.

Day of Surgery

► *Andrew has spent the night on a couch in the hospital lounge. They give me a sedative very early in the morning. He watches them wheel me toward the elevator. He tells me later there are tears in his eyes and a giant lump in his throat as I wave goodbye to him. I don't remember it.*

I remember only glimpses, sounds, feelings: the elevator doors opening as my bed is wheeled in; the cool, white tile of the operating room; the feel of cold metal instruments being placed on my body; a steady, rhythmic beating.

"Is that my heart?" I ask no one in particular.

"Yes," says a distant voice. Nothing is familiar.

"Cathy?"

Ah, at last. It's my doctor's voice. My wonderful, wonderful doctor.

"Hiiii," I smile. He laughs.

I think of a joke: "I hope you're more coherent than I am." But I can't make my mouth say the words.

I feel, rather than see, lots of motion.

People begin to surround me. I fall into a very deep sleep.

An orderly will take you to surgery on a wheeled bed. You will probably have to part with your mate now as most hospitals do not allow visitors in the surgery area. When your specialist is ready, the anesthesiologist will start your medication. You will feel drowsy rather quickly.

The Operating Room

Many patients are semiconscious when they are brought into the operating room. It is a cool, tiled, sterile, brightly lit room with lots of equipment. And it should be. The instruments and machines are there to protect your life. The coolness and sterility are necessary to prevent infection. Nevertheless it is a frightening, sobering sight for most of us.

There will be many gowned and masked people in the operating room, including your specialist, the anesthesiology team, and several surgical nurses. They will greet, reassure, and perhaps joke with you as you are gently moved onto the operating table. Things may seem unreal or dreamlike. The surgical team members then begin their work, placing monitoring devices on your chest and preparing you in other ways for surgery.

Three types of anesthesia may be used: general, regional, or local. *General anesthesia,* most often used during microsurgery, induces unconsciousness and numbs the areas of the brain that feel pain. You will have no memory of the surgery. Your blood pressure and respiration will be slowly lowered to appropriate levels for the surgery. An injection of a drug such as sodium pentothal induces immediate unconsciousness for a short period of time. Once you are asleep, a tube is inserted down your windpipe. Nitrous oxide gas is then administered through this tube to keep you unconscious during the surgery. The side effects of general anesthesia include nausea, headache, and dizziness, and are sometimes experienced for several days after surgery. Very rarely (in about 1 out of 10,000 to 20,000 cases) severe complications such as paralysis or death may result from this type of anesthesia.

Sometimes regional anesthesia such as a *spinal* or *caudal,* where the patient remains conscious, may be used. With a spinal, the anesthetic is injected into the spinal canal and produces numbness in a general area of the body, such as above or below the waist. For some types of fertility surgery or cesarean births, the lower half of the body from the waist to the toes is numbed. Recovery from a spinal is faster than with general anesthesia. A *caudal,* similar to spinal anesthesia, is injected into the air spaces of the spinal column. The nerve endings leading to the legs and pelvic area are numbed. Some patients have headaches for a day or two after regional anesthesia.

Once anesthesia is administered, the surgery begins.

Recovery

► *I heard someone calling my name from far away. I had to travel many miles to reach that voice. It seemed I had been away for the longest time, and it was hard to come back.*

The voice became louder. Now I could speak myself and answer, "Yes, I'm here."

After surgery you are brought to the recovery room to regain partial consciousness, although you may not have a clear memory of it. The recovery room nurses will check you frequently to note your progress. One nurse will call your name and stay with you until you respond. Your surgeon may also speak with you briefly. You are then brought back to your room to regain full consciousness. Your spouse, friends, or family can stay with you here.

The hours following surgery are usually foggy, surreal ones. You'll doze on and off for several hours as the anesthesia slowly recedes. You will also be given pain medications, which often make you groggy. When you are fully awake, it will be surprising how much time has elapsed since your surgery. It may be hard to believe you were "gone" for so long!

THE CATHETER A catheter (a slender plastic tube) will be in serted in your urethra during surgery. While you are unconscious and immobile, your urine passes through this tube into a plastic pouch. If inserted properly it should not cause any pain. When you are awake and able to move, the catheter is removed. This is usually a quick procedure but may cause some mild discomfort.

GETTING BACK ON YOUR FEET Most postop patients are urged to walk immediately after regaining full consciousness. Although it is stiff and painful to move, you can shuffle along slowly and you will be encouraged to walk the short distance to the bathroom. A bedpan will be unnecessary, although sitting on the toilet usually causes noticeable pain around your incision at first.

There may be a measuring cup attached to the toilet bowl to catch and measure your urine. This is sometimes done for a few days to compare the fluids leaving the body with the amounts entering intravenously. Because the preop enema has cleansed your bowels, it will be three or four days before you have a bowel movement.

THE IV EQUIPMENT During surgery you will be placed on intravenous (IV) fluids to provide hydration and nutrients. The fluids flow from a bottle or bag suspended from a wheeled pole about six feet high called an IV stand. Plastic tubing, with valves to control flow, is attached to the bottle. A needle at the end of the tubing is inserted into an arm vein near your wrist and securely taped in place. For many infertility surgeries, an IV hookup is used for several days to administer medications that ease pain and inhibit scarring and infection. You can push the IV stand ahead when you walk.

THE PAIN

► *The pain after surgery is different from any I've experienced before. It hurts, but is good rather than sick pain. My body is slowly knitting itself together and healing.*

► *When I was in the recovery room, a voice came from far away and said, "Cough, dear." When I did, the pain was worse than I had ever imagined. It felt as if a fistful of burning matches had been dropped on my abdomen. The voice came to me once more and said, "Cough again, dear," and I was so drugged that I did.*

Later in the day I discovered that with fluids constantly dripping in through the IV, I had to urinate frequently. When I asked for a bedpan the nurses said it was time to walk to the bathroom. I couldn't believe they were serious. They were, and I passed out half way there. The bad part was that in order to get back to bed I had to walk there! What amazed me was how much easier it was the second time. By the third trip it was a relative snap.

As these two stories illustrate, patient's reactions to pain vary tremendously. Usually pain is severe for a few days after pelvic surgery, and then diminishes each day afterward. You are given pain medication immediately after surgery, and your specialist will leave orders with your nurse for periodic injections for the next several days.

Everyone has a different tolerance for pain, and all of us react differently to drugs. After the first day or two after surgery, you can decide how much medication you need and how often to request it. It does take awhile for the drugs to work, so allow enough time to let them take effect.

CHECKING VITAL SIGNS While you are hospitalized, your vital signs (temperature, blood pressure, and pulse) will be checked every four hours to ensure you don't develop an infection or other postop complication. This necessary procedure prevents you from sleeping more than several hours at a stretch and adds to postop fatigue.

PHYSICIAN'S ROUNDS Your specialist will visit you on morning rounds each day and perhaps in the evening after office hours. In addition he or she will be in contact with your nurses to check your postop progress.

Second Day

► *I felt a searing, burning sensation across my abdomen the morning after surgery. Lying perfectly still the pain was least noticeable, but any movement that put tension on my abdominal muscles greatly magnified it. I noted the pressure dressing on my abdomen. An IV was running into my arm, and a catheter was draining my bladder. Though I'd awakened briefly several times during the night, this was the first time I felt lucid and coherent. Eclipsing all other thoughts, including those of the pain, was my concern about my future fertility. I was still a bit too dazed to obtain that information. After awhile a medical student came in who had attended the surgery. She assured me that my remaining Fallopian tube had looked normal.*

► *It is painful and difficult to sit up, even with the hospital bed adjusted to the highest position. It feels as if a metal band has been wrapped around my belly and is being tightened mercilessly. I put my feet on the floor. A nurse helps me stand up. I feel weak and want to crawl back in bed.*

"C'mon," she coaxes, "you're doing great."

Reality sets in as you begin your second day. The full impact of surgery is hitting your body, and it may feel like you've gone ten rounds with a prizefighter. It hurts to cough, laugh, walk, or even talk. To keep your lungs clear of fluids you must periodically roll onto your side and cough. To regain your strength and reactivate your metabolism, you should walk every few hours. Both these movements will be uncomfortable or painful. The tubes used during general anesthesia often cause a sore throat and hoarseness for a day or two. You've also lost sleep as nurses check vital signs and change IV medications.

MEALS For the first day or two after pelvic surgery you'll be served a "clear" diet of fruit juice, broth, and jello. Although this is bland and unexciting cuisine, it is important to restart the digestive process gently after surgery. Eating rich foods too soon can result in painful intestinal cramps. In fact many patients who have pelvic surgery experience severe gas pains, which subside as the air remaining in the abdomen passes out.

After a day or two most patients can tolerate solid food. Your menu will be changed to a "soft" diet of oatmeal, boiled eggs, custards, cottage cheese, and similar foods. About the fourth or fifth day after surgery, a full diet of meats, starches, fruits, vegetables, beverages, and desserts is introduced. By this time you're ready for hearty fare!

HEARING ABOUT YOUR SURGERY AND FERTILITY PROGNOSIS

► *"Only about 50 percent of women who've had endometriosis go on to have children," my doctor says, watching me closely.*

"Why?"

"No one knows."

I've stopped listening. I'm looking at my husband. I'm waiting for him to say something.

He doesn't but looks back at me.

"I don't like those odds." I can't think of anything else to say. I'm really thinking how worthless I am, how infertile, how barren.

The silence lies between us.

"Well, if that's the way it is," I mumble.

I'm really thinking, "Hell, I've beat tougher odds than this. I still think I can do it."

I don't dare say it. I don't think anyone will believe me, let alone encourage me.

That night I lie awake a long time. I keep thinking about that 50 percent chance.

What are numbers? You just don't get 50 percent pregnant. How do you translate statistics into feelings? It would be easier to get through this if I knew it would eventually lead to a pregnancy. But I don't.

I can't think of anyone to talk it over with. My roommate has two kids; the nurses just smile and plump my pillows; my mother wants to be a grandmother; my doctor tells me there are no guarantees. And I can hardly face my husband.

Patients are either semiconscious or unconscious during their surgeries, and most are eager to hear about the operation. Your doctor will review the surgery and perhaps give you a prognosis for a future pregnancy, often in terms of a percentage.

You may be relieved to hear positive news that brings hope for a biological child. Depending on the nature and degree of damage, your chances for pregnancy may be as high as 50 percent. The problem may even have been minor and easily corrected. On the other hand, you may be surprised and stunned by a poor prognosis. You may hear discouraging statistics, perhaps in the 10 to 30 percent range, or that your fertility problems were worse than any of you had anticipated.

We feel vulnerable after surgery, and a poor prognosis can be overwhelming. It is frightening to discuss surgery in any case, and feelings of confusion, anger, and fear are natural. It helps to lean on your loved ones and continue this dialogue with your specialist throughout your hospital stay.

Third Day

► *I noted a marked decrease in my incisional pain. It was easier, though still painful, to move, cough, or laugh. I took oral pain medicine, rather than injections. Less relenting were my feelings. Though I could be distracted from them by visitors or staff, I cried when alone in my room, feeling an almost cosmic sadness and vulnerability. Yet I was relieved that everyone seemed to think I would be able to have a baby. Though painful, I resumed a lot of my normal activities: eating, grooming, getting up, and walking around. I found the pain to be worse at night. As much as I needed rest and sleep, I did not sleep well, despite the medications.*

By the third day, you will be accustomed to the hospital routines of shift changes, vital signs checks, mealtimes, visiting hours, and the quiet nights when the hospital sleeps. Many patients, however, report an emotional crash of tears and depression around this time. Around-the-clock monitoring has taken its toll and adds to overall exhaustion. Expect this letdown and remember it won't last forever. Curl up with a favorite book, call a loved one, or just cry. Above all love yourself for your courage, strength, and spirit.

VISITORS AND PHONE CALLS

► *I speak with my grandfather on the phone. "Are you all right?" he asks. He doesn't ask me if I'll be able to have children now as so many others do. I feel better as I talk to him. He always makes me feel special and loved for who I am. Our conversation is good medicine. I feel stronger.*

Love and laughter are among the strongest healing medicines. Both during your hospitalization, and later at home, you'll need reassurance and emotional support. Surround yourself, physically and emotionally, with caring people. Ask those who make you feel happy and loved to visit or call.

Listen to your body as well as your heart. Do you need solitude, company, or rest? Patients' moods and strength vary each day after surgery. You may feel terrible today but stronger and eager for visitors tomorrow. Pace yourself on the number of visitors and calls and be honest with others about your wishes. Remember that you are in control: You can request the hospital switchboard to hold your calls for any part of your stay.

YOUR POSTOP BODY

► *I was both fascinated and saddened by my incision. It was graphic proof I had been cut open and forever changed. Just as I felt different inside, my body would always look different outside.*

Major pelvic surgery requires a "bikini" incision, of two to four inches across the lower abdomen below the pubic hairline. After surgery the incision will be covered by a large bandage or dressing taped across your abdomen. When this dressing is removed on the second or third day, you will see your incision: a bright red, straight, narrow line. It fades with time but will always be visible. The incision is secured both underneath with sutures and on the surface with either knotted stitches of a fine material that resembles fishing line, or "staples," surgical clips that are easily and painlessly inserted and removed. These temporary stitches will be removed in the next day or two. Your abdomen will be puffy and bloated regardless of your preop fitness. It will be some time before your figure returns to its previous shape.

From today on you can probably take a sponge bath or a shower and shampoo your hair. A nurse will wrap protective plastic around your abdomen to keep the incision dry. Although you are given plenty of "open-air" hospital gowns, most patients quickly tire of them. Today you can change into cheerful, comfortable clothing. Many patients find that a hot shower and change of clothing lift their spirits considerably. It is satisfying to return to daily grooming routines and do things for yourself.

Many patients are taken off the IV on this day or the next. If intravenous medication is still occasionally needed, a "heparin lock" may be used. This device consists of a needle with a plug or "port" attached. The needle is inserted in a vein near the wrist and the device is securely taped in place. Whenever needed an IV or hypodermic needle can be inserted into the plug to administer medication. You will now have more mobility and can walk without the encumbrance of an IV stand.

Fourth or Final Day

► *The fourth day was easier physically. I took fewer pain medications. The feeling of being physically wounded lessened, but I still felt very fragile. I was also aware of healing and realized how far I'd progressed since the surgery.*

Over the next few days you will often be asked whether you've had a bowel movement or passed gas. These events indicate your intestines and bowels are again functioning normally. By now some of us are no longer self-conscious with such personal questions in the hospital setting, although others still feel embarrassed.

Most patients are released between the fourth and sixth days after surgery, but each recovers at her or his own pace. Your specialist will review and discuss your progress daily.

Postop Instructions

On the day of your release, your specialist will have specific instructions for gradual resumption of physical and sexual activity. Among other things, you will be told to get plenty of rest, sleep, and nutritious foods, given a prescription for pain medication, and asked to schedule a postop visit four weeks later.

Every surgeon is concerned about the patient's first few weeks after discharge. Indeed, many patients underestimate their weakened condition and push themselves too hard. This can result in exhaustion or complications. You have been cut and sutured through several layers of skin, muscle, and connective tissue. It will take a full six weeks for these layers to heal fully. Be careful not to strain your incision by lifting even fairly light objects, climbing more than a few stairs, or even pushing a vacuum cleaner!

Convalescence

► *Coming home was bittersweet. I cried as I walked through each room, touching familiar things. It was good to be home and I felt safe again, but I had so many intense, contradictory feelings! I wanted to be taken care of, pampered, and cuddled. I felt wounded, weak, and helpless yet proud of myself, changed, and different from everyone else. I was stronger and much older than I had been just a week ago.*

Since major surgeries require a convalescence of four to six weeks, make arrangements with your employer for a six-week leave of absence. Return early only if both you and your specialist agree this is wise. Your homecoming may be an emotional one. In less than a week, you've experienced a great deal of physical and emotional stress.

Hospital routine often lingers and may take several days to fade. For a few nights, you may wake up routinely for vital signs checks. Your feelings of weakness and dependency may also continue for awhile.

First Week

This week should be completely devoted to the rest needed for healing from the surgery, regaining strength, and making up for lost sleep. Take both a morning and an afternoon nap, get plenty of sleep each night, and keep visitors and calls to a minimum. You will probably feel weak, and walking will still be slow and stiff. The pain should subside by the end of this week, although you can continue taking the prescribed medication. Pamper yourself with warm baths; good novels; hearty, nourishing meals; and other treats.

Second Week

This week is usually an easier one. Your strength should be steadily returning, although rest is still important. Try to take at least one nap each day and get a good night's sleep. You may now want to encourage visiting from friends and family to pass the time and lift your spirits.

Third Week

By the third week you should feel more like yourself. Some postop patients now feel restless, even a bit stir crazy. "Confinement" (between hospital and home) is four weeks old, and many active people are now eager to get back into the world. If you feel up to it and your specialist agrees, start taking very short walks or outings. Ask a friend to accompany you. On your first try slowly walk a short block and then back home. Don't walk a half mile your first time out or overdo any activity.

Fourth Week and Beyond

During your fourth week, you'll visit your specialist for a postop checkup. He or she will examine your incision to ensure that it is healing properly, note your general progress, and perhaps order a blood count to check for anemia.

If all is well, your convalescence will draw to a close. Your specialist may still want you to refrain from full physical and sexual activity for another week or two. You may now want to discuss the next stage of your infertility treatment. If not, schedule another appointment in a month or two for this purpose.

Over the next several weeks, your energy and strength should slowly return. Your body, mind, and spirit, however, have been sorely taxed. Many postop patients tire easily for several months after surgery, and it may take awhile to resume a busy life-style. One woman found it took six months before she could again complete a 50-minute aerobic and toning exercise routine. Be patient with your healing and praise your body for a strong, steady recovery.

Evaluating Your Hospital Stay

As a patient and consumer of medical services, it is important to provide feedback to hospital administrators and your specialist about the overall quality of your care. Consider writing a letter after your hospital stay commenting on both the positive and the negative aspects of your experience. It is unfortunate that few people praise the many positive contributions of hospital staff, though most are quick to complain about questionable or poor health care. A letter of commendation will give deserved thanks and recognition to these dedicated, hard-working health care providers.

If you are dissatisfied with your experience, write a letter to the chairperson of the hospital's board of directors. You can obtain his or her name and address from the hospital switchboard. Be concise and thorough in your assessment of the problem, and try to give some suggestions about what could be done to improve the situation in the future. A copy of your letter will be forwarded to the appropriate hospital personnel. Most health care providers appreciate constructive criticism, and changes may be made that will benefit future surgical patients.

The Effect of Your Surgery on Your Loved Ones

► *Everything seemed to look and taste gray. I would return to the desk every ten minutes and ask for news, but the answer was always the same. The operation was still in progress and nothing beyond that was known. Time seemed to stand still and I felt trapped in an existential hell where time had no meaning.*

All kinds of fears began to prey upon my mind. The surgery was only supposed to take an hour. By the time the third hour had come and gone with no word, I feared that cancer had been discovered and her doctor was trying to remove it to save her life.

This chapter has focused primarily on the fears, needs, and experiences of the surgical patient. A few words, however, should be said about the effects of your surgery on your loved ones.

Fertility surgery is usually scheduled after a diagnostic workup. Your specialist will probably have some idea of the problem but can only estimate the length of the surgery. Operations commonly run over their estimated time when the problem is worse than originally thought or other areas need attention. There may also be a delay before surgery begins. Fertility surgeries may take from one to five hours.

For the groggy or unconscious patient, the actual time in surgery is a blur. It is an eternity, however, for your mate, family, and friends. Time drags until they hear that the operation is over and you are all right. Afterward your specialist may meet with your mate to discuss the procedure and prognosis. Your partner then carries that weight until you are alert and ready to hear it.

Your absence will be keenly felt at home, and your countless daily efforts sorely missed. Once you're back, you'll still be partially disabled. All told the household will be in turmoil for several weeks. Try to remember how difficult this is for your family. Expect everyone to feel exhausted and "stressed out" before this is over!

Children

Couples experiencing secondary infertility, or those with a stepchild, are concerned about the effect of surgery on their children. (For a discussion of secondary infertility, see Chapter 6.) A toddler will only vaguely understand that you will be having an "operation." Children from 2 to 5 years old are noticeably affected by your absence and disability and the disruption of household routine. Older children are better able to understand your surgery.

It is important to be calm and reassuring with any child. All kids worry about their parents' health and the stability of their family life. One pediatrician advised a mother to compare her surgery to repairing the car!

► *When our car is not working right, we take it to the garage to be fixed by a mechanic who understands about car problems. I have a problem with my body. My doctor, who understands about such things, is going to fix my problem at the hospital. I will be fine and can call you on the phone every day! I'll be back home in a few days.*

Arrange loving, stable care for your child while you are in the hospital. Grandparents can fill this role nicely, and close family friends or relatives are also great baby-sitters.

Together your family will decide on how much visitation, if any, is appropriate. You may prefer to wait until intraveneous medications are stopped because some children are frightened by this sight. Older children can usually cope with hospital atmosphere and will be relieved to see you.

Many hospitals encourage family visits and allow children on most floors. Some provide a visiting lounge on postop floors, furnished with comfortable sofas, chairs, and pictures. Ask in advance about your hospital's policies and visiting hours for kids.

You can, of course, chat on the phone every day. You may want to call your child in the morning to tell him or her of your progress and then again in the evening to say goodnight.

Suggestions for Helping Your Family Cope

The key to helping your family cope with your surgery is to take good care of yourself. Your outlook and attitude will affect everyone else in the family. Chapter 7 offers many suggestions for maintaining good health. In addition, the following hints are offered:

- Plan ahead! Arrange in advance for help while you're hospitalized to relieve your spouse. Many friends and relatives will offer their assistance. Ask them to help with child care, household tasks, shopping, errands, chauffering, and meal preparation for four weeks after surgery.
- Leave your home neat, clean, and organized. Together with your mate make sure the housework and laundry is done, bills paid to date, and freezer and cupboards stocked before you leave. Prepare and freeze a dozen or more dinners. You can make a double recipe of most soups, stews, casseroles, and pasta dishes and freeze half. Whether wife or husband has the surgery, this will be a great help during the first two weeks of convalescence.
- Fix up your bedroom for a comfortable, enjoyable convalescence. You'll be spending lots of time resting in your bedroom for the first several weeks after surgery. If there isn't a phone there, make sure the nearest one has a cord long enough to reach. You may also want to set up a portable TV or radio. One woman even put a cooler in her room and stocked it with juices and ice water, so she wouldn't have to go downstairs for a drink! Also stock up on lots of reading.
- If your car has a stick shift, plan to borrow one with an automatic transmission for a few weeks. After pelvic surgery, most specialists prefer that you not drive a car with a manual transmission during your convalescence because it places additional strain on your legs and pelvis.
- Have realistic expectations of yourself and your family. Your hospitalization and convalescence will be a difficult, stressful time. If possible your mate should arrange a week of leave after your surgery to supervise the household routine and recover from the experience. Otherwise be sure to arrange enough help so you can have complete rest during the important first week of convalescence.

Repeated Surgeries

► *The second try at major surgery was very different from the first. I had been through it all before and was five years older. It was harder to keep my spirits up, and I took longer to convalesce.*

Because medical problems such as endometriosis or adhesion formation can and do recur, some patients undergo more than one major surgery. Others require one or more follow-up laparoscopies for in vitro fertilization or to check scar tissue formation.

Many of us can "psych up" and summon the energy to get through one operation. Additional surgeries often seem physically and emotionally overwhelming, and the chances for pregnancy decrease with each attempt. Still some couples pursue surgery again, hoping to be one of the fortunate, successful minority. If you should repeat major surgery, keep yourself physically and emotionally fit.

Emotional Aftermath of Surgery

For most patients, major surgery is a powerful event, a time of transition and intense feelings. Afterward many experience a wide range of emotions from relief, exhilaration, and triumph to apprehension, sadness, and depression. Some feel significantly different, changed, or older.

In the days following surgery, it is not unusual to find yourself cheerful or sociable in the morning and tearful or withdrawn a few hours later. Some patients become depressed once they are home. The hospital experience is over and their repressed emotions now surface in a safe and loving environment.

This emotional aftermath may remain for months or years. For some fertility surgery is like a pregnancy loss, and many remember and retain feelings about this experience throughout their lives. Others look back at their surgery as a turning point, a time when infertility came into focus and was confronted with positive, determined action. Some will ultimately experience a successful pregnancy, and others will adopt a child or opt for a child-free life-style. In any case surgery was another important step in their resolution process.

CHAPTER 6

Secondary Infertility

► *Our son Joshua, almost four and a half, was unplanned, unexpected, and conceived while I used a diaphragm. When he was a year old, we tried to conceive again. At first we discovered a luteal phase defect after I stopped nursing him. Recently I had surgery to remove the endometriosis that stole my fertility in one short year.*

Secondary infertility is the inability to conceive and birth another child after one or more successful pregnancies. The incidence of this condition is increasing as couples defer childbearing into their thirties and forties. This inability to conceive second or subsequent pregnancies now accounts for more than half of all fertility complaints. Although similar to primary (first-time) infertility in some respects, this problem raises its own unique issues.

Ironically the couple's first pregnancy may have been achieved without difficulty, or accidentally while using contraception. Conversely that pregnancy may have been the miraculous result of years of frustrating tests, drug therapies, or surgeries.

► *So it began again—thermometers, fertility drugs, exams. After six months and no pregnancy, the old feelings arose again. Even worse, we knew what was ahead. My poor body screamed, "Please don't cut me open again!" Feel-*

ings of inferiority washed over me with surprising force, magnified by the second pregnancies of our baby-sitting coop members —those fertile ladies I so gratefully befriended after Jenny's birth.

Some couples, who were lucky once, decide to challenge infertility a second time. They love being parents and, despite the familiar miseries that lie ahead, are willing to try again. Those painful infertile feelings, which probably receded with the triumph of a first pregnancy, usually resurface with surprising intensity. Their first infertility experience has also consumed a great amount of time, energy, and patience. To add to this "stress level," they've just spent an exhausting year or two parenting a small child, a tiring albeit welcome experience.

Neither Fertile nor Infertile

► *After eighteen months I finally conceded. Something was terribly wrong—again. Who could I talk to? My fertile friends? They were pregnant again within six months of trying. My infertile friends? I am humbled by the courage of those unable to conceive or carry to term and too ashamed to complain about my problem. After all, I did have one successful pregnancy. I feel all at once greedy, selfish, inadequate, and isolated. I decline invitations to baby showers yet again.*

One woman describes secondary infertility as "neither fish nor fowl." Indeed many people find this problem a contradiction in a couple with one biological child. With one success visible in their firstborn, friends and relatives find it difficult to accept the couple's subsequent infertility. They reason that if pregnancy happened once, it will easily occur again. Many couples are also astonished to receive a diagnosis of secondary infertility, particularly if their first pregnancy was easily achieved.

Primary infertiles usually offer little sympathy. They often resent couples who have successfully birthed a child, have little patience with their fertility complaints, and believe their own pain would disappear if only they could bear one child.

Regardless of how many children they have already birthed, victims of secondary infertility often feel anguish when their fertility is impaired and grieve for their babies not yet born. Both fertiles and primary infertiles find this pain difficult to comprehend. Each group may view one success as enough, leaving the secondary infertile couple isolated and without support.

Social Pressures

► *Well-meaning people advise, "Don't wait too long to have another" because "one is so lonely." Maybe they didn't hear me say I was infertile? Maybe they don't believe me?*

Often I've found myself apologizing for being the mother of an only child.

Secondary infertiles, as well as those who intentionally have only one child, usually encounter tremendous social pressure to enlarge their family. They are often told and may even believe that a threesome is not a complete family, and that they have an obligation to provide a sibling for their firstborn. They find themselves defending their decision or, if infertile, explaining and perhaps apologizing for their one-child family.

They also hear the insensitive remarks common to infertility. Along with advice on how to conceive, there may be curiosity about the ease or difficulty of their first pregnancy. Secondary infertility also prompts its own unique comments such as, "Be grateful for the one you have!" "Relax! If you had one, you'll have another!" "What are you waiting for? Give this child a brother or sister!"

It is good to remember that families don't need four, five, or six members to be real or complete. There are families of varying sizes in this world, some biologically related and others not. When asked why you have only one child, consider a direct reply such as: "We'd like more, but we have a medical problem." This will usually stop the questions. Your honesty may also encourage others to discuss their own challenges and create opportunities to share support and empathy.

With strangers or insensitive acquaintances, however, complete honesty may not be appropriate. If someone indicates your child and asks, "Just the one?" a simple answer of "Yes" is all that is necessary.

The Infertile Family

► *Having had no problem whatsoever conceiving our son, my husband and I wanted another child right away. We were 24 and 25 years old at that time.*

After about a year I saw an infertility specialist and underwent the whole workup. My tubes were severely damaged from an old infection I never knew existed. At that time he performed a laparotomy, opening the ends of the tubes. Six months later, still no baby. During that time, my husband and I divorced. While this wasn't our only problem, I'm sure the feeling I could never have another baby made me quicker to leave him.

► *I experienced the entire range of emotions that come with infertility. In some of my blacker moments, I even forgot I had a child because he forced me to deal with fertile people. We cannot escape the fertile world. Our son looks forward to Christmas parties with relatives. He attends a nursery school where almost monthly someone else becomes pregnant and I envy her excited glow.*

Infertility often affects communication, sexuality, and stability in even the most secure marriages. Financial troubles usually add another worry. Infertility testing, medications, surgery, or counseling costs add up quickly. (See Chapter 3 for a discussion of the economics of infertility.) In addition to these expenses, the couple is already incurring the considerable cost of raising a child. There are bills for pediatricians, child care, clothing, and nursery schools. Parenting itself undoubtedly strains a marriage, so secondary infertile couples face two challenges at once!

Their child, sensitive to parents' feelings and moods, is also affected by infertility but cannot fully understand why. Mom and Dad, aware of this confusion, are trying to cope with their own feelings and function in a fertile world. Having one child has immersed them in a milieu of playgroups, nursery schools, birthday parties, baby showers, and holiday gatherings. Reluctant to discuss their problem with others, infertile parents find these events awkward, although their child is usually eager to attend parties that include young children.

Household routines are sometimes disrupted if complex testing, surgery, or in vitro fertilization are necessary. Additional help may be needed with housework, errands, and child care if a parent is hospitalized or convalescing. Such variations in routine can be frightening to a small child, who fears for Mom or Dad's safety and the security of the family.

Sensing that their child is literally irreplacable, parents may become extremely protective of an only child and unusually fearful that he or she may be hurt or killed. These feelings may ease somewhat after grief for lost fertility is completed. It helps to realize that many couples share similar fears as they pass their reproductive years. "Letting go" as a child grows and seeks independence is difficult for most parents.

A Sibling or Not?

► *There were times when I felt guilty for feeling so obsessed with getting pregnant. Maybe I should have been thankful for having one beautiful, healthy baby when there are couples who have none. But I felt the same feelings childless women have when they see "pregos" or a newborn, and I also felt incredibly guilty for my son, who will never have siblings.*

Social pressure aside, many parents want their child to have one or more siblings. When infertility prevents an addition to their family, guilt or a sense of failure often result. And many children around the age of three ask why they can't have siblings like their friends do.

It is usually wise to be honest with children, in discussions appropriate to their ages, about fertility problems. Explain that you are sorry that you cannot have another baby just now, but you are still a family.

► *We'd all love to have a little brother or sister for you. Maybe we'll have another baby some time, and maybe we won't. Whatever happens, we're lucky to have you! We love each other and are a wonderful family of three.*

Keeping in touch with your child's feelings is important. Children need reassurance that grief and sadness do subside and, most importantly, that they are in no way responsible for their parents' unhappiness.

Some couples initiate adoption proceedings to enlarge their families. In such cases an honest discussion about adoption can ease your child's worries during the waiting period and the first few months after your new child's placement. (See Chapter 17 for a discussion of adoption.)

If pregnancy is not likely or possible and adoption is not the right choice for you, try "extending" your family with close friends or relatives.

Coping as a Family

► *We've learned patience and acceptance because of it. My son amazes me with his awareness of what is going on. He has never asked why he has no sisters or brothers; he knows because we discuss it. As for Joshua, he's only four; the best is yet to come!*

It's important not to let infertility dominate your lives. Take advantage of the flexibility of a family of three and set aside time for fun and enjoyment. Perhaps this is the year for that first trip to Disneyland or a camping trip in the mountains. In time you'll decide whether to be content with one child, pursue further medical treatment, or adopt. It helps to share your sadness as a family, while maintaining a positive attitude that you will persevere and triumph together.

CHAPTER 7

Taking Care of Yourself

► *The first three and a half years of my treatment were aimed at inducing ovulation. For the last year and a half prior to conception, however, I was ovulating regularly, and all other tests on my husband and myself were normal. In thinking back on that time, I realized what was different:*

- *I was getting regular aerobic exercise twice weekly for one hour.*
- *I had weekly massages.*
- *I incorporated the use of "positive visualization."*
- *I gave up my longtime addiction to chocolate and coffee after hearing about the connection between caffeine and fibrocystic breast disease. I thought this couldn't hurt, since I had cystic ovaries.*

I was living a healthier life in general. At the time I became pregnant, I had come closer to accepting that it would never happen. Previously it had been an all-consuming obsession, a stage in infertility I feel is hard to overcome.

I believe in a holistic approach to infertility treatment, including stress awareness and reduction, nutritious diet, regular aerobic exercise, and a foundation of hope (along with the moments of despair) if pregnancy is indeed possible. Because infertility is a very stressful life crisis no matter how it is resolved, taking care of one's self physically and emotionally can benefit everyone.

It is common to equate infertility with disease or poor health. Although organic problems may be detected in either partner, infertility itself is not always an indication of disease, illness, or weakness. Other signs of physical well-being, such as a strong cardiovascular or nervous system, a normal hormonal balance, or overall strength and stamina often exist in the presence of infertility.

The physical, emotional, psychological, and social pressures of infertility, however, often affect our well-being and influence our life-style. Through anger or depression, we may punish ourselves with sleepless nights, infrequent or nonexistent exercise, or indulgence in heavy, fattening junk foods. Over time these habits can take a toll, creating a syndrome of depression and poor health.

You can avoid this pitfall by taking good care of yourself physically, emotionally, mentally, and spiritually. Such a life-style fosters a healthy self-image. Infertility then becomes a personal challenge to tackle as a strong, determined, and healthy person, rather than a weak and passive victim of life.

Nurturing Physical Well-Being: Diet and Exercise

A healthy, nutritious diet is essential throughout your life. During times of extended stress it is especially important to provide the protein, carbohydrates, vitamins, and minerals that your body needs to maintain optimal physical and emotional well-being.

If you are trying to conceive during infertility testing, you must also think about nourishing your baby during early gestation. Three critical weeks of fetal development may pass before pregnancy is confirmed. Even if you are unable to become pregnant right away, good nutrition now is an investment toward a safe pregnancy, a healthy baby, and a stronger Mom later. Many experts recommend preparing your body for a full year before trying to conceive.

What Is a Healthy Diet?

A well-balanced daily diet includes the four major food groups: milk and dairy products; fresh fruits and vegetables; breads, cereals, and other whole grains; and meat, fish, and poultry. A balanced vegetarian diet, consisting of complete amino acids (created through combined plant proteins such as corn and beans), along with essential vitamins and minerals, is another alternative.

Salty, fatty, and overprocessed foods are best kept to a minimum or not consumed at all. They provide only empty calories, high in fat or sodium and low in essential nutrients. Red meats and fried foods are also high in saturated fats and contribute to increased cholesterol levels. Try substituting fish, poultry, and leaner meats for hamburgers and steaks.

Also try to avoid foods high in refined white sugar or sucrose. Besides contributing to tooth decay and perhaps diabetes and hypoglycemia, sucrose creates an artificial "high." Unlike other natural sugars such as lactose and fructose, which are absorbed slowly by the body, sucrose enters the bloodstream almost immediately. The body must then produce excessive amounts of insulin to process it, which over time exhausts the pancreas. After the sucrose is burned off, your blood sugar level plunges, creating a feeling of letdown or depression.

Many of us consume refined sugar products all day, driving our pancreas ever harder to process all those doughnuts, candy bars, sodas, cookies, and other sweets. In addition, many prepared foods such as catsup, mayonnaise, salad dressing, snack crackers, granola bars, and cereals contain excessive amounts of sucrose in the form of corn sweeteners. Try substituting fresh fruit, which contains fructose, for refined sugar products. Read labels carefully before buying any product, and try to eat as much fresh, unprocessed food as possible.

It is also important to eat whole grains in the form of cereals, breads, pasta, beans, rice, and other grains. White rice and refined flour products, as well as many cereals, lose their outer husk or bran in the milling process. This outer shell provides many vitamins and minerals, and roughage to move food quickly through the body.

Americans consume a largely refined grain and high fat diet, have one of the highest rates of colon cancer in the world, and spend millions of dollars on drugs to alleviate constipation. Daily bowel movements will occur naturally with a regular exercise program and a diet that includes whole grains. If you feel the urge to snack, try popcorn instead of candy, potato chips, or other empty calorie junk foods.

Weight Control

Many Americans are obsessed with weight loss and constantly seek the miracle diet or consume pills to shed unwanted pounds. Nutritionally unbalanced or "crash" diets, which strain the metabolism and nervous system, are detrimental to both emotional and physical health. Diet pills are harmful drugs, stimulants that affect the body's chemical balance. Weight should be controlled naturally with regular exercise and a proper diet.

Caffeine, alcohol, artificial sweeteners, nicotine, and other drugs are also harmful to the body. They deplete vitamins, may cause numerous health problems, and should be avoided if you are trying to conceive.

Exercise

► *For me exercise was a positive counterpart to the negative self-images of infertility. Although my body would not easily conceive, it did respond beautifully to a daily workout. I felt and looked better physically at 34 than I did at 21!*

Many experts believe that engaging in regular aerobic exercise is as critical to our health and well-being as consuming a nutritious diet. Such exercise strengthens the cardiovascular system, tones muscles, and sheds fat. Exercise is also a great outlet for tension. In short it is a perfect antidote to the physical and emotional demands of a stressful world. For these reasons, it is wise to consider a lifetime commitment to regular aerobic exercise—appropriate to your age, stamina, and overall health—both during your infertility and afterward.

Many people are unsure of what aerobic exercise is, or how it differs from the calisthenics of their high school or college days. *Aerobic* combines the Greek words for *air* and *life* and is defined as "living or thriving on oxygen." Essentially, aerobic exercise is a consistent, uninterrupted workout that demands steady exertion of the body's muscles and cardiovascular system for 20 to 25 minutes. Full deep breaths, which nourish and sustain the working muscles with oxygen, are inhaled and then expelled in a *comfortable* breathing pattern. You are not out of breath and should be able to carry on a conversation. Jogging, jumping rope, "power walking," swimming, dancing, cross-country skiing, and bicycling are all popular aerobic exercises.

Before starting an aerobics program ask your physician whether you should have a complete physical examination and review any medical conditions such as obesity, heart problems, or injuries. Long-distance running, for example, can exacerbate knee, foot, and shin injuries.

If you have a sound heart and good overall health and are not seriously overweight, you should be able *gradually* to master an aerobic routine of 20 to 25 minutes duration over a few *months*. Don't try to do the entire routine the first few times. If you feel out of breath while exercising, slow to a walk and finish your time. Don't stop suddenly and "surprise" your heart! You should find your endurance and strength increasing with time. *To maintain fitness, a minimum of three, and a maximum of five, aerobic workout sessions per week is recommended.*

An additional 20 to 30 minutes of stretching and toning work on your arms, abdomen, thighs, hips, calves, and buttocks is also recommended during each exercise session. Modify your workout if you have back, leg, foot, or neck problems. Trained instructors can suggest alternate positions for exercises that are painful or uncomfortable. Many gyms also offer classes in "low" or "nonimpact" aerobics, which minimize the pounding movements on the legs and feet.

Choose an aerobic activity you enjoy. If you'd rather exercise alone, design an individual program. There are several resources for the individual exerciser. Physicians specializing in sports and fitness medicine can help you plan an aerobics program, as well as treat any exercise-related problems. In addition there are many good aerobic exercise books and videotapes.

Make exercise a special part of your day. This is a time to renew your body and mind, strengthen your heart and lungs, shore up damaged self-esteem, and vent a lot of nervous energy! This conditioning is also an important asset for the arduous and demanding job of pregnancy, birth, and early parenting if you should conceive, the physically exhausting first year of parenting if you adopt, and the stresses of everyday life if you remain child-free.

Maintaining Emotional Health: Reducing and Coping with Stress

► *I conceived four months after stopping clomiphene therapy. I was ovulating with it for a year and a half before. I'm not sure exactly how or why I got pregnant after five years, but I believe that weekly massage helped relax my body and perhaps affected my hormonal problems. I don't mean to imply that people should "just relax" and they'll get pregnant. But if a hormonal problem is involved, perhaps relaxation techniques could help bring your body back to balance.*

In conjunction with medical treatment, some women and men have used such techniques as massage, meditation, visualization, acupressure, and chiropractic to reduce the stress of infertility. Many find that massage releases tension that has concentrated in certain parts of their bodies. Others state that quiet periods of meditation put worries into perspective and calm the spirit. There has been increasing evidence that visualization of a healthy, healing body is effective in treating many diseases, including cancer.

Acupressure is an ancient Eastern healing technique that applies gentle pressure to key energy points or "meridians" to restore balance within the body. Chiropractic treatment involves manual adjustment of the spinal column, rather than drugs or surgery, to relieve nerve pressure that can result in back and neck pain, menstrual cramps and irregularities, and tension headaches. According to chiropractic theory the nervous, endocrine, and muscular systems are closely aligned and strongly affect each other. A pinched nerve or misaligned vertebra may influence normal bodily functions.

If you decide to see a chiropractor, or any practitioner of stress reduction techniques, *exercise the same care and caution as in choosing any health care professional.* This field has its share of unethical or incompetent practitioners, and the buyer must truly beware.

Some infertility patients who employ one or more of these stress reduction techniques *in addition* to medical treatment report a resumption of ovulation, a greater overall sense of well-being, and sometimes even pregnancy. Do these alternative methods really work? Can they offer a "cure" for infertility? Would those pregnancies have occurred anyway? No one knows.

Our specialists are the first to admit how little we really know about infertility. It is important to remember, though, that no person or method can guarantee a pregnancy. In our anxiety to become pregnant, it is easy to pin all hope on our specialists or alternative health treatments. If we can keep a perspective that there are no guarantees or cure-alls, stress reduction and relaxation techniques can ease the inevitable pressures of an infertility challenge.

Coping Techniques

The social pressures of infertility, exemplified by the comments of others, the pregnancies of friends and relatives, and the occasions that celebrate children are often unavoidable. However their impact on your self-esteem and marital relationship can be alleviated.

To cope with thoughtless or insensitive remarks from relatives, friends, and acquaintances:

- Consider discussing your infertility with those you trust, perhaps a favorite sister, cousin, or grandfather with whom you have been close. Confiding in someone you love and trust can ease your tension and give them a positive way to help.
- Be selective in whom you confide. Not everyone will understand your feelings or treat you in a sensitive, caring manner. Sometimes temporary physical or emotional distance from insensitive or thoughtless people is helpful.
- Together, decide what is private information about your infertility, and what each of you is comfortable sharing with others. Discuss ways to handle comments and support each other when such situations occur.

Stick together at gatherings you suspect will be awkward, don't make your mate field questions all alone. When relatives offer unsolicited advice, put your arms around each other, smile, and say, "We're taking care of this ourselves, thank you." Tell a nosy neighbor or aunt that you do not wish to discuss the subject. Or use humor with each other and curious relatives.

- Ask well-meaning friends not to bring up the subject again. Explain what a difficult time this is and ask for their support. They may think their interest is a form of caring and concern. Being honest about your reactions to their remarks will help them understand your feelings. If possible, suggest ways they can help you.
- Give the following letter, reprinted from Ann Landers' column, to persistent friends or relatives. It may ease your discomfort and educate them at the same time:

DEAR ANN LANDERS:

Please print this list of requests for relatives and friends of infertile couples. It could save a lot of tears:

1. Please don't call every month and ask if I'm pregnant. If I were, I'd be so excited I'd shout it from the housetops.

2. When your kids misbehave, don't ask me if I want them—or worse yet, if I would like to buy them. I'd pay anything for a couple of kids—well-behaved or not.

3. At the next baby shower, don't say to me, "You'll be next." I've been disappointed so many times that I have a terrible feeling that I will never get pregnant. It's all I can do to look at baby clothes without crying.

4. Don't make us feel guilty when we buy some luxury by telling us you can't afford such things because your kids cost so much to raise. We'd gladly give up all the extras to have children like yours.

5. Don't put us down for considering adoption and say you couldn't honestly love someone else's child. The minute that adopted baby is in my arms, he will be the same as my very own.

Ann, please find space to print this. There are thousands of childless couples who have to put up with these insensitive and hurtful remarks every day.

P.S. My husband and I have spent five years and thousands of dollars on tests that have shown no reason for our infertility. We are now waiting to hear from one of many adoption agencies.

—MAYBE SOMEDAY

DEAR MAYBE: Let me know when you get pregnant or a good news call from an agency. I'll rejoice with you!

Coping with the pregnancies of other women, especially those you know and love, is often painful for both sides. Your mixed feelings of envy and happiness are natural and understandable; in turn, your pregnant friend may fear her success will jeopardize your friendship. She may also feel ambivalent about her pregnancy if it was unplanned, or anxious if she has previously miscarried or been infertile. There are also mixed feelings when infertile friends become pregnant or adopt. Because this experience has bonded you, it is natural to feel abandoned or alienated when they become parents.

Some ways to handle this situation include:

- Try to have an open exchange of feelings—although envy as well as happiness often surfaces—about how the pregnancy is affecting your relationship.

► *During this period one of my pregnant friends took the time to call and spend time with me. She shared her pregnancy with me in a compassionate, sensitive way. The more I wanted to withdraw and hate myself, the more she stayed with me. Another pregnant friend did not, and we are now casual acquaintances. Because of the caring of my one friend, I am able to share joy in other people's pregnancies and babies. I know that their ability to have or not have babies will never make me either fertile or infertile.*

- Record your feelings. One infertile woman kept a journal of her feelings during her best friend's pregnancy. Her attitude slowly changed toward her friend and the unborn child. The newborn, once a source of pain, became a treasured and precious baby to her.

- If an honest expression of your feelings will be either ineffective or inappropriate, decide how much, if any, contact with pregnant acquaintances you want. As you move toward resolution, this jealousy usually subsides. You can again share a pregnant friend's happiness, aware that parents do not have idyllic lives and may sometimes envy you!

- If you want to, decline baby shower invitations and simply send a gift. You are entitled to your feelings and no apology or explanation is necessary. After resolving their infertility, some women feel comfortable attending baby showers and may even host one for a pregnant friend.

Holidays, those seasonal reminders of our infertility, are often difficult to live with. However you can soften the "holiday blues" in some specific ways:

- Accept that holidays are often awkward, stressful occasions for everyone, and especially for an infertile couple. Instead of denying sadness or anger, set aside time to express your thoughts to trusted friends or a counselor.

- Choose which holiday events to attend and stay only as long as you feel comfortable. You may want to schedule several "escape events" that you know will be enjoyable. For example, some infertility support groups plan child-free festivities during the holidays to laugh, celebrate, and commiserate.

- You are already a family of two. Why wait to create your own traditions? Perhaps you can go skiing during Christmas, or plan a romantic getaway on Mother's Day or Father's Day to renew your commitment.

- Seek others who find holidays difficult. Perhaps you have neighbors who live far from relatives and would welcome company during Christmas or Chanukah. Seniors are also often alone on holidays, and hospitals, nursing homes, and churches welcome volunteer help on these days.

Special Coping Suggestions for Stepparents

In this era of widespread divorce and remarriage, many women and men are creating "blended families" composed of newly married partners and children from previous unions. The stepparent role, a difficult one in any case, can intensify the emotional stress of infertility. The partner without a biological child is often pressured by his or her family to produce "a child of your own," and many couples want to have at least one child together. In any event your partner was once fertile with his or her ex. You are not—at least for the present. Jealousy, anger, and a sense of inadequacy toward your mate and his former partner are natural reactions.

► *When I began my infertility treatment, I was already a stepmother to 3- and 7-year-old daughters who lived with us. While most of the time I felt more fortunate than other infertiles in that I had an opportunity to be a mother, the times that their biological mother visited heightened my pain. I was essentially ignored by the girls. This seemed to emphasize my lack of fertility—reminding me that I was not their "real mother."*

You can soften these feelings by acknowledging that even though your partner did reproduce with someone else, he or she still grieves for the infertility of *your* union. Mourning together for your unborn baby is an important process.

Although stepchildren cannot replace a child of your flesh, a close and loving relationship with them enables you to experience a different, but nonetheless important, kind of parenting.

► *Seven years later, the 3-year-old who is now 10, still lives with us, and feels as much mine as my 1-year-old daughter whom I carried inside me for nine months.*

Special Coping Suggestions for Single Women

► *I could not find a specialist in Los Angeles who was willing to administer artificial insemination by donor to an unmarried woman. Everyone who hears I am single and infertile criticizes me for my desire to parent a child alone.*

► *I went through several years of unsuccessful inseminations. It was so difficult to find emotional support. Most people think gay women have no business being mothers anyway, and even among the gay community there are those who are opposed to pregnancy or uneducated about infertility. So I felt alone and very frustrated with my infertility.*

A growing number of single women, who hear the reproductive clock ticking in their mid- or late thirties, are choosing to have a child through artificial insemination by donor. This decision is usually criticized by friends and relatives, and a single woman must constantly justify why she wants and deserves to be a parent. She may also be refused treatment by disapproving physicians or clinics. If she encounters a fertility problem or a pregnancy loss, her experience is usually not acknowledged as the "real problem" that a married woman might suffer. Single women also hear all the tactless infertility comments, plus a few others: "You're not getting pregnant because there's no man in your life," or "Just get married and then you'll get pregnant!"

A single woman doesn't have to contend with a resistant or uncooperative partner and can make unilateral decisions. At the same time, no one else has a vested interest in her fertility and she lacks a support system to provide empathy and interest. This isolation, along with the negative reactions of others, often leads her to suppress her emotions and inhibits the resolution process.

Infertility also occurs among gay women couples who wish one partner (or both) to bear a child. Like single women, they may be criticized for their wish to parent, and since most infertility and adoption literature is geared toward middle-class, heterosexual, married couples, it's difficult for single and gay women to find peer support. Times are slowly changing, though, and more is being written about single women and infertility. In addition, some women's health clinics and other referral agencies facilitate or encourage support networks.

Fostering a Positive Attitude

► *I recognized that I had gained the strength through all this to handle pregnancy or childlessness. I think a great deal of my earlier motivation was my fear of not having children and being labeled a barren and therefore useless woman.*

Now I knew that I had proven myself to the only person who mattered—me. I had gone all the way—the workup tests, surgeries, and fertility drugs. I had faced it and carried it through.

I realized that it wasn't necessary to have a baby to prove my worth or value as a woman. Pregnancy would be a welcome gift, not a mandatory condition for my survival. Either way I would go on.

I tried to plant positive seeds in the relationships and projects with which I was involved. I kept busy and, when I was depressed, reminded myself that it was normal to feel low about infertility. Even fertile people get the blues; they're part of living!

Together with physical and emotional well-being, a positive mental outlook enables you to face infertility with determination and strength. The importance of psychological and emotional support cannot be overemphasized. To laugh, cry, and talk with another infertile woman or man provides the "reality check" to get you through a tough day. Keeping a journal during this experience is therapeutic and provides a valuable, timely perspective on a challenging time.

During your infertility it is also important (and healthy!) to keep in contact with children. They provide a very different and often refreshing world view. One woman suggests clocking some "baby hours" with the infant of an understanding friend or relative. This may ease your ache for an infant and provides a welcome respite for weary parents. The wails and constant demands of an infant or toddler also bring parenting into a realistic perspective. If caring for infants is too painful, try including your friends' or siblings' older children in some of your activities. The ages of 7 to 12 are golden years when kids require little physical care and are delightful, fun-loving companions.

Humor is also an essential part of mental health and an invaluable ally during an infertility struggle. Without the ability to laugh at adversity it would be difficult to face any problem. Infertility has its share of absurdities, enabling us to laugh as well as cry.

► *Misery not only loves company but also develops a sense of humor. It's extremely comforting to know that other husbands besides mine practically pack their bags when their wives get their periods. My husband isn't the only one who gets chided by friends for "shooting blanks" or for not "figuring out how to do it yet." I don't even feel so strange anymore for having made love once when I had strep throat and poison oak and he had a broken leg, simply because it was "that time of the month!"*

Think about the "props" of infertility: thermometers, BBT charts, drugs, postcoital tests. Or the awkward situations: four close friends who call the same day with news of their pregnancies; a nagging grandmother-in-waiting who looks at you and sighs a lot; and the out-of-town visitors who show up on your fertile night. When all else fails, find someone who understands and trade infertility humor.

Your physical, emotional, and mental health can lead to a path of healing and personal growth. After assessing and treating your medical problem and pursuing an appropriate resolution, you can again take control of life by channeling your energy into avenues of fulfillment and achievement. Accepting a challenging promotion or beginning further studies can provide a welcome and positive diversion to a stubborn fertility problem. Professional counseling may also clarify personal and collective goals.

PART II

Diagnosis, Causes, and Treatment of Infertility

PROLOGUE

Human Reproduction

Knowledge of the anatomical and hormonal aspects of human reproduction is critical to a patient's understanding of the diagnosis, causes, and treatments of infertility. A basic and highly simplified discussion of the female and male reproductive systems, as well as the miraculous processes of ovulation, spermatogenesis, and conception, follows.

The endocrine system, composed of a group of glands that secrete essential chemicals called *hormones* directly into the bloodstream, plays a critical role in orchestrating all body processes, including human reproduction. The endocrine glands—the thyroid, parathyroid, adrenals, pancreas, pituitary, hypothalamus, testes, and ovaries—ideally work in unison to maintain health. Hormones such as thyroxin, adrenalin, and insulin (secreted by the thyroid, adrenals, and pancreas) influence various metabolic processes.

Endocrinology, the study of this intricate system, has become an important part of infertility treatment. Scientific advances in the past decade now enable measurement of subtle hormonal changes and treatment for many abnormalities. More couples with infertility problems caused by hormonal imbalances can now be helped.

The synchronized interaction of the hypothalamus, pituitary, and sex glands direct sperm production, ovulation, and early pregnancy. This is accomplished by the "sex" hormones estrogen, progesterone, prolactin, and testosterone, which are produced in both men and women.

The *hypothalamus* plays a critical if not fully understood role in directing hormonal activities. Located under the cerebral cortex of the brain, this important gland controls appetite, body temperature, and emotional integration. The hypothalamus receives signals from the brain, and has the crucial function of translating these messages to other reproductive organs.

In response to chemical and electrical messages, the hypothalamus secretes gonadotropin-releasing hormone (GnRH) into miniscule blood vessels that travel to the pituitary gland. Communication between the hypothalamus and pituitary is necessary for ovulation or sperm production (spermatogenesis) to occur. It is known that extreme stress can disrupt hypothalamic activity, which may temporarily stop its signals to the pituitary and cause menstrual irregularities or even cessation of menses. (This reaction, however, is more common in adolescents and not considered a likely cause of infertility.)

The *pituitary* gland also plays a crucial role in male and female reproduction. Less than half an inch in diameter, it is located at the base of the brain, between the eyes. This tiny gland synthesizes and stores several hormones necessary for normal functioning of the ovaries and testes.

The Female

Unlike the male's, a woman's reproductive organs are contained entirely within her body (see illustration).

The *vagina,* the passage between the vulva and the uterus, is between three and five inches long. It is a muscular organ, that normally has a fairly acidic environment with a pH of about 4.5. The penis is enclosed within the vagina during intercourse and ejaculates semen into it during male orgasm.

The *cervix* is the narrow base of the uterus, which connects it to the vagina. Its tiny opening, the *os,* allows semen to enter and menstrual fluid to depart. The cervix contains many tiny glands that secrete different types of mucus throughout the menstrual cycle.

The *uterus* (also called the *womb*) is a pear-shaped, muscular organ lined with endometrial cells and can stretch to many times its normal size to accommodate a growing fetus.

The *Fallopian tubes* (or *oviducts*), each about four inches long, are attached to the uterus at the narrow end of each tube. Their wide, trumpetlike openings hover near each ovary. Tentaclelike projections called fimbriae protrude from the ends of the tube, surround the ovary, and retrieve the egg. The tiny inside passage of the tube—a mere 1/70 inch in diameter—is lined with cells that secrete lubricating fluids, as well as hairlike cilia that beat more than 1000 times per minute. The cilia and lubricants propel the egg toward the uterus.

The almond-sized *ovaries* are attached by stalks to the uterus. These female sex glands, which ideally release at least one mature egg (ova) each menstrual cycle, also produce estrogen and progesterone hormones.

THE FEMALE REPRODUCTIVE SYSTEM

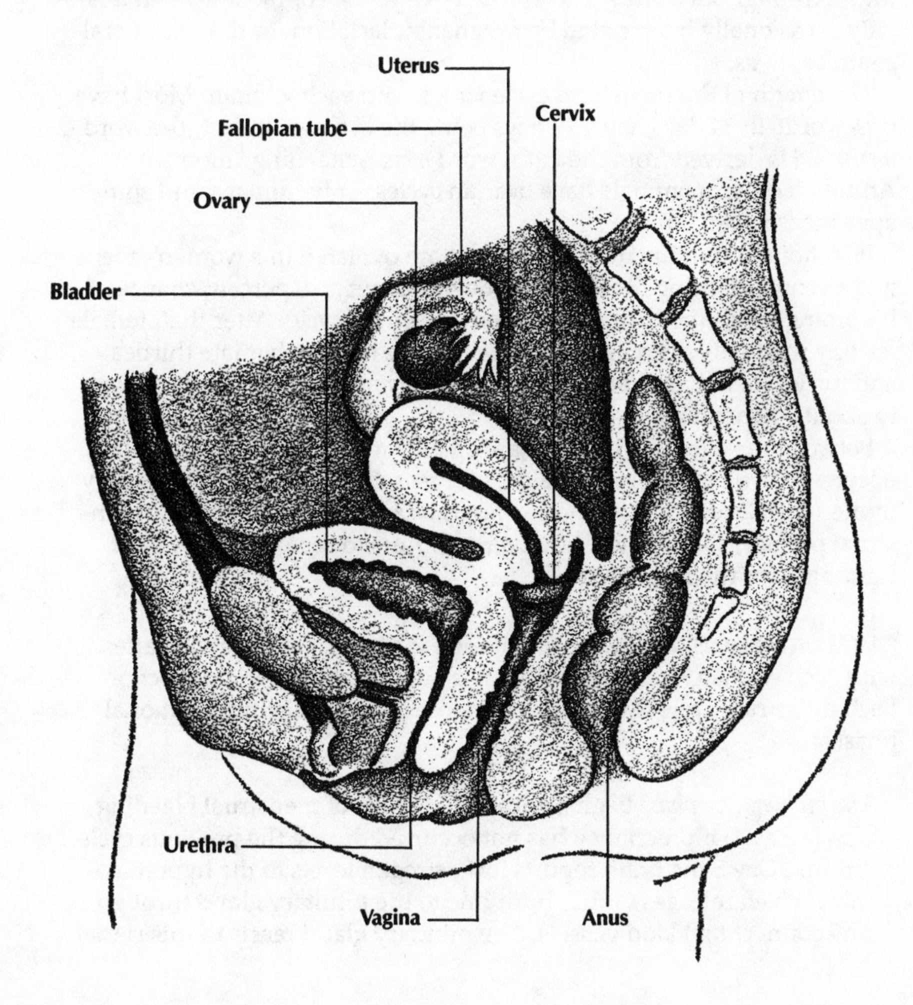

The Menstrual Cycle

A female infant is born with 1 million to 2 million immature ovarian follicles called *oocytes.* Many oocytes disintegrate throughout childhood during the *atretic* process. When menstruation begins (*menarche*), most girls have about 400,000 ova. Although the atretic process continues throughout life, most women retain enough viable follicles to ovulate about 400 eggs during their reproductive years.

At around 9 years of age, the hypothalamus "wakes up" in young girls, initially secreting gonadotropin-releasing hormone (GnRH) only at night. Activity gradually increases until GnRH is released about every 90 minutes around the clock. The ovaries and pituitary react to this signal, release other hormones, and the first menstrual period occurs.

Ideally the hormonal cycle that results in ovulation and menses continues throughout a woman's reproductive years. For most women it is only occasionally interrupted by pregnancy, lactation, or the use of oral contraceptives.

The length of the menstrual cycle varies with each woman. Most have cycles of 26 to 34 days, with 28 days being the average. In fact, the word *menstrual* is derived from the Latin word *mensis* meaning "month." Although other mammals have ovarian cycles, only humans and some apes menstruate.

It is thought that the most fertile eggs are ovulated in a woman's teens and twenties. During these years, she has about a 20 percent chance of becoming pregnant during any given menstrual cycle. After that, female fertility markedly decreases with age. As she reaches her late thirties and forties, her chance for pregnancy during any given cycle decreases to about 8 percent.

Between the ages of 45 and 55, a woman simply "runs out" of viable oocytes to ovulate and begins a gradual cessation of fertility, commonly termed the *climacteric* (technically *menopause* refers only to the last menstrual period.) The ovaries, however, continue to secrete low levels of hormones for the rest of her life.

PHASES OF THE MENSTRUAL CYCLE Although the length of the cycle varies with each woman, a 28-day cycle is used as an example in this section. Each menstrual cycle is normally composed of four distinct hormonal phases:

1. *The proliferative phase* begins with the first day of menstrual bleeding (Cycle Day 1) if pregnancy has not occurred during the previous cycle. Around Day 5 the brain reports low estrogen levels to the hypothalamus, which releases GnRH hormone to the pituitary gland through tiny connecting blood vessels. The pituitary gland reacts to this signal

and secretes large quantities of follicle-stimulating hormone (FSH) and smaller amounts of leutinizing hormone (LH).

Responding to increased FSH levels, about 1000 oocytes begin to develop within each ovary. Through Day 8 the developing follicles continue to absorb FSH and produce more estrogen. One fluid-filled follicle, among the first to develop and usually the largest of both ovaries, soon becomes dominant. In response to the increasing estrogen levels, the pituitary slows FSH production. The smaller follicles cannot absorb enough FSH to maintain themselves and die off. The dominant follicle absorbs all available FSH and continues estrogen production.

During this phase increasing estrogen levels cause the endometrial lining to thicken. Between Days 11 and 13, hundreds of cervical mucus glands secrete a clear, stringy, "sperm-friendly" mucus and the os dilates slightly.

2. *Ovulation.* Within the ovary, the dominant oocyte (called the Graafian follicle) has fully matured in its sac. The egg is surrounded by two layers: the innermost zona pellucida, surrounded by the cumulus oophorus, which gives the ovum a cloudlike appearance. The ovum's chromosome count has been reduced to 23. When fertilization occurs, the sperm will contribute another 23 chromosomes, giving the embryo the normal human chromosome count of 46.

   By Day 13 estrogen has been maintained at peak levels for about 48 hours. This prompts the hypothalamus to increase GnRH production, which signals the pituitary to release a surge of LH hormone. When the LH surge has been maintained for about 24 hours, the wall of the follicle disintegrates and the surface ruptures. The miracle of ovulation occurs as a fertile ovum, only 1/150 inch in diameter, is released from the ovary.

   The egg floats away and is retrieved by the tentaclelike fimbriae of the Fallopian tube hovering near the ovary. The fimbriae grab the cumulus layer and propel the egg down the tube.

3. *The luteal or secretory phase.* Responding to the LH surge, the ruptured follicle sac undergoes a "leutinizing process." Its cells enlarge and absorb a yellow pigment called lutein, which the body manufactures from cholesterol. It is now called the corpus luteum, a Latin phrase meaning "yellow body," and has the critical job of producing a great deal of progesterone and smaller amounts of estrogen for 10 to 14 days. Successful implantation and early pregnancy depend on this perfectly balanced hormonal production.

   During the luteal phase, the progesterone surge will trigger other important changes:

- LH production in the pituitary will be suppressed.
- Basal body temperature will slightly elevate, the basis for "documenting" ovulation through BBT charting.
- The endometrium will change to a "secretory state." Its lining will soften and prepare for implantation and nourishment of a fertilized embryo. The character of these postovulatory endometrial cells differ markedly from those of the proliferative phase.
- The cervical mucus glands shift back to producing thick, opaque secretions, and the os shrinks. These changes discourage the entry of sperm or other foreign matter.

If pregnancy does not occur within about 14 days after ovulation, the corpus luteum ceases its hormonal production and disintegrates.

4. *Menstruation.* The endometrium responds to the decreasing progesterone level and releases chemicals called prostaglandins. Uterine contractions and perhaps cramps result, menstruation begins, and the endometrial lining is shed. Bleeding, which varies from light to heavy among women, usually lasts from three to seven days. Most women lose only about two ounces of blood.

   During menstruation, the brain senses lowered estrogen levels and signals the hypothalamus to secrete GnRH to begin a new cycle.

The Male

The male reproductive organs, pituitary, and hypothalamus compose an intricate and complex system that ideally manufactures, stores, and ejaculates millions of sperm. As with female reproduction, hormonal, environmental, or physical factors can easily upset this balance and cause male fertility problems.

A boy begins the sexual maturation process of puberty at around 12 years of age. Over the next three years, his body manufactures large amounts of male testosterone hormone, which dramatically increases his sex drive, stimulates body hair growth, deepens his voice, and, together with other hormones, produces mature, fertile sperm.

In addition to testosterone mature males produce other hormones common to both men and women, such as FSH, LH, prolactin, and estrogen. These hormones are secreted on a continuous basis; thus a man does not have a "cycle" comparable to ovulation, and sperm are constantly regenerated throughout his lifetime. Although sperm counts may decrease with age, men do not experience a cessation of fertility comparable to female menopause.

The Male Reproductive System

Unlike the female's, a male's reproductive organs are housed outside his body in the *scrotum*—a pouch with several inner linings and an outer layer. It has two chambers and hangs behind the penis and away from the body (see illustration.)

Each chamber contains a testicle, blood vessels, nerves, and a spermatic cord that transports the sperm. Since sperm production is inhibited by body temperature, this ideal external location keeps the testicles cool (about 94° F).

Each *testicle* is about two inches long and an inch in diameter and weighs about an ounce. Its primary function is to produce sperm and testosterone hormone. Each testicle contains convoluted *seminiferous tubules,* which would measure several hundred yards if uncoiled. Within these tubules are the immature sperm cells, which are sensitive to fevers, viruses, and other illnesses. For this reason sperm production may be slowed or halted during sickness.

THE MALE REPRODUCTIVE SYSTEM

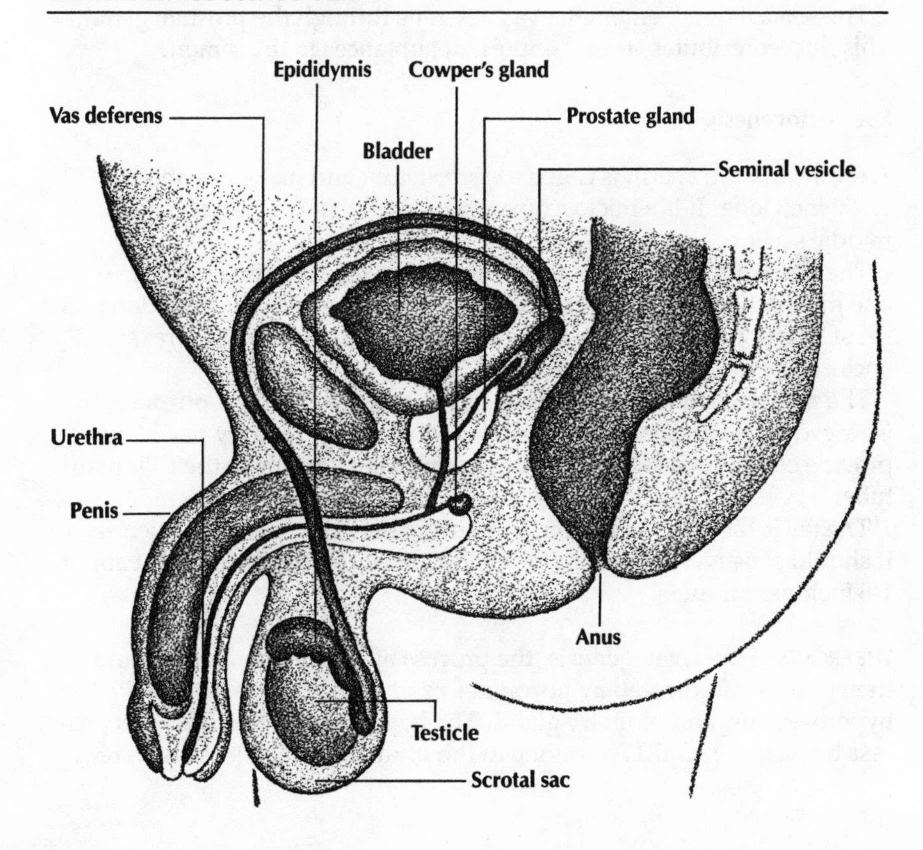

The *Leydig cells,* located throughout the testes, produce testosterone hormone, which is emptied into the veins and carried into the bloodstream. These cells are not as heat sensitive as sperm cells, so a man's sex drive, voice, or hair growth are usually not affected by illness or fertility problems.

Each testicle is connected to a long, complex, and convoluted system of ducts, which are critical to sperm maturation and transport. The *epididymis,* the first section of this duct system, is only about 1/125 inch in diameter and occupies about an inch of space in a tightly coiled "C" shape. Unwound it would measure nearly 20 feet.

The epididymis is connected to a *vas deferens,* two sturdy ducts that enter the body on either side of the abdomen. Each vas moves up through the groin and the anal canal, behind the bladder, through the prostate gland, and into the urethra. This is the duct that is cut during male sterilization (vasectomy).

The *prostate gland* lies in front of the seminal vesicles and surrounds the urethra. It is about an inch and a half in diameter and generates much of the milky, alkaline seminal fluid. This gland sometimes enlarges later in life, which may cause problems with urination.

The *seminal vesicle* enters the vas deferens through the prostate gland. This duct contributes several important subtances to the semen.

Spermatogenesis

A fertile, mature sperm is called a *spermatozoon* and measures about 1/500 inch long. It is a microscopic, wiggly cell that consists of a head, middle section, and tail.

The head of the sperm measures about five microns (one micron = one millionth of a meter). It contains the father's genetic information in a set of 23 chromosomes, as well as important enzymes, which are enclosed in a cap called the *acrosome.*

The middle section is quite small but serves an important purpose. It is ringed with bands of mitochondria, which act as "battery packs" to provide continuous energy for the sperm's long journey to the Fallopian tube.

The tail is the longest section, measuring between 30 and 50 microns. It should constantly flagellate, propelling itself toward the ovum at about 1/8 inch per minute.

THE PROCESS Spermatogenesis, the process of sperm manufacture and transport, is coordinated by hormones produced by the testes, hypothalamus, and pituitary gland. The hypothalamus initiates this process by releasing GnRH hormone to the pituitary, which in turn secretes

FSH and LH, also known as interstitial cell stimulating hormone (ICSH). Testosterone is produced in response to these hormones; the germ cells within the testes begin to mature and develop tails; and the sperm are released into the epididymis. At this stage they are unable to swim or fertilize an egg. They are moved through the epididymis through rhythmic contractions (peristalsis). During this process, which takes 10 to 14 days, they become both motile and fertile.

The sperm next enter the vas deferens and are again advanced by muscular contraction. During this journey, the prostate gland contributes enzymes, magnesium, phosphates, and zinc to the semen. The seminal vesicles contribute prostaglandins and fructose sugars, which provide fuel to sustain motility. All these substances help the semen coagulate upon ejaculation and then reliquify 5 to 25 minutes afterward in the vagina.

The combination of seminal fluid (98 percent) and sperm (2 percent) make up the *semen*. One-third of this fluid is stored in the last portion of

DETAIL OF SPERM

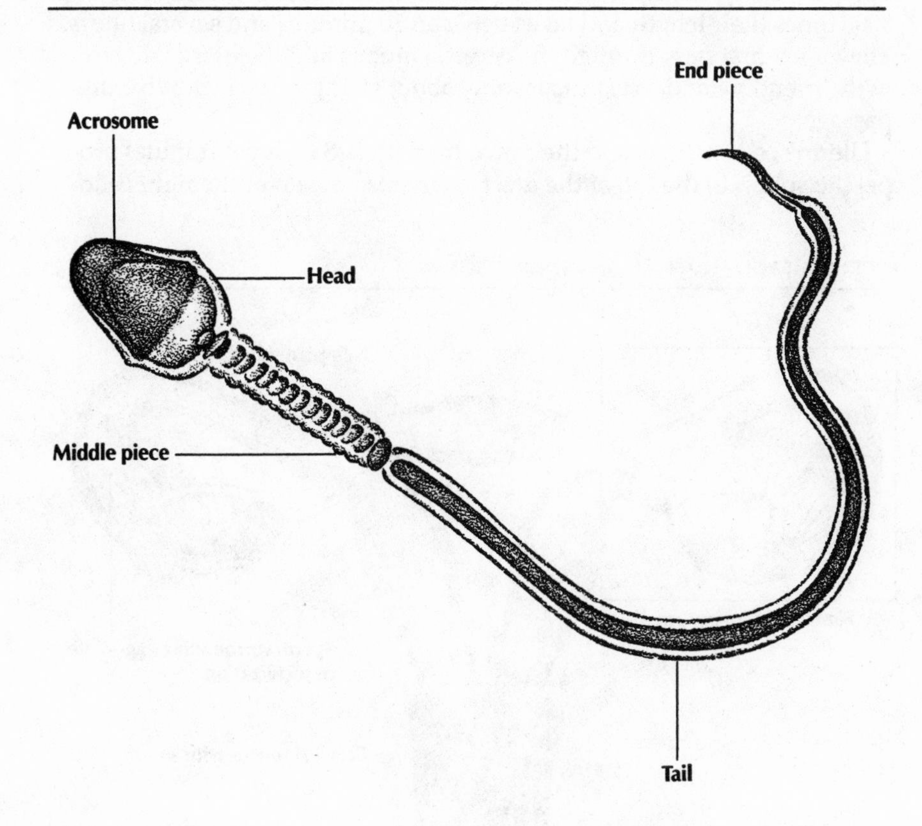

the epididymis; the rest awaits orgasm within the vas deferens. When the male is sexually excited, the semen enters the *urethra,* a tube that runs through the penis, and is ejaculated into the vagina during orgasm. Because the urethra also carries urine, during erection the body cleverly engages a muscle that blocks urine flow.

The entire process of sperm production and transport takes about 90 days. Although mature sperm die if not ejaculated within a month, the continuous release of FSH and LH hormones results in constant sperm regeneration. The new sperm are transported to the vas to replace the old.

Conception and Pregnancy

Minutes after ejaculation, the semen jells into a thick, white substance that reliquifies within the vagina about 20 minutes later. The sperm then begin the long journey to the Fallopian tubes, a distance that is nearly 3000 times their length and takes between 30 minutes and several hours. They must first pass through the cervical mucus into the uterus. Even with "friendly" midcycle mucus, only about 400 sperm will survive this passage.

Uterine contractions and their own motility (1/8 inch per minute) propel the sperm to the top of the uterus, where some enter the right Fallo-

JOURNEY OF EGG AND SPERM AND THEIR UNION

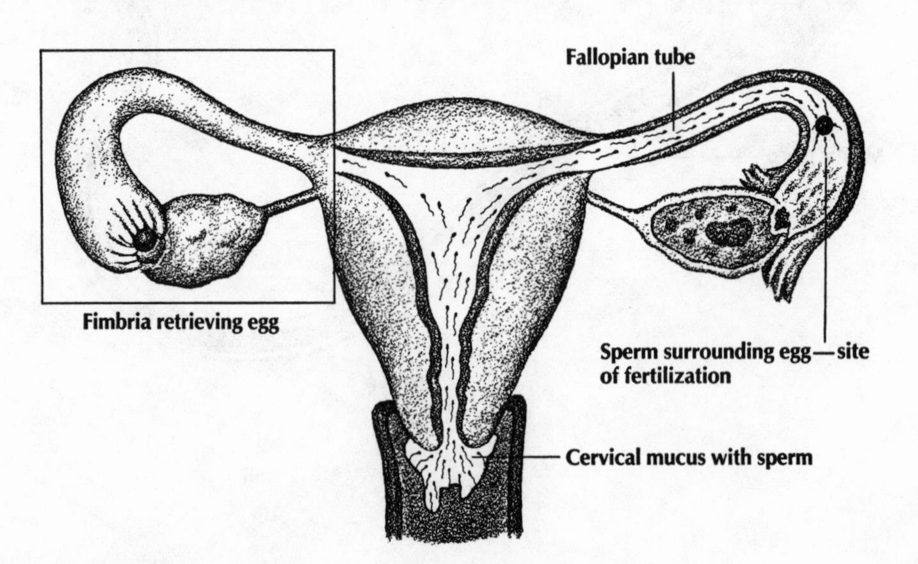

pian tube and others the left. They are stored in cavities in the Fallopian tubes and are slowly released a few at a time. More will be lost as they swim through the tubes searching for an ovum. Out of an initial ejaculate of perhaps 100 million sperm, fewer than 200 will reach the egg as it floats down the Fallopian tube.

During this journey the sperm gradually go through capacitation, a mysterious process that enables them to penetrate an ovum. The sperm's cap is slowly worn away to release its enzymes. One of these, hyaluronidase, helps forge a path through the outer layer of the egg; another enzyme, acrosin, breaks down the inner layer so a small slit, only large enough for a single sperm, can be made.

Conception occurs as the sperm fertilizes the egg, their chromosomes blend, and a chemical reaction occurs that reseals the membrane. This is nature's way of preventing other sperm from entering and creating an embryo with three or more sets of chromosomes.

The fertilized egg is now called a *zygote* and contains 23 chromosomes from each parent. Over the next few days, the zygote divides in half and then quickly divides twice more. At the eight-cell stage it moves to the uterus, and, if it successfully implants, produces HCG hormone for the next three months. This sustains the corpus luteum's production of progesterone and estrogen until the placenta can take over. HCG hormone can be detected in an early serum pregnancy test.

A great deal of early pregnancy loss occurs naturally within the body. In general only about 31 percent of ova exposed to fertilization will survive to a term birth. In older women this percentage decreases.

Clearly many conditions must be ideal in both partners for pregnancy to occur and proceed to term. Physiological problems that may cause female, male, or combined infertility, as well as current medical treatments, are discussed in Chapters 8 through 16.

CHAPTER 8

The Female Infertility Workup

► *I began my infertility workup with mixed feelings. It was a frightening, uncertain time. I couldn't get pregnant, and we didn't know why. I also felt inadequate because I wasn't fertile and angry that tests were necessary. Yet starting the workup also felt like a positive step. I wanted to know what was wrong and try to fix it. It gave us both a sense of control and brought us closer together.*

Most women become pregnant within a year of starting to have unprotected intercourse. A couple therefore should attempt to conceive for at least this long before beginning intensive infertility testing. Earlier testing, however, may be appropriate for women over 30, for those with known medical problems that will affect fertility, or when anxiety is affecting the couple's marriage or either partner's self-esteem.

Such factors may include irregular menstrual cycles or painful menses (not relieved by antiprostaglandin medication), past history of pelvic inflammatory disease (PID), exposure to DES, prolonged use of an IUD, or endometriosis. (These problems are discussed in Chapters 10 and 11.)

When first attempting pregnancy, a general discussion about fertility with your internist or gynecologist is often helpful. The physician can provide useful information about average conception time, indications of ovulation, cervical mucus changes, chances of miscarriage, and perhaps instructions about basal body temperature (BBT) charting.

Consulting an Infertility Specialist

If pregnancy does not occur within a year, your physician should order a semen analysis. Gynecologists may also perform the postcoital test and perhaps hysterosalpingogram (described below). If these tests indicate a problem, or if infertility continues, it is wise to consult an infertility specialist. In most cases the patient need not repeat basic workup tests already performed as those results can be transferred to the specialist. Selecting a specialist who is medically competent and emotionally supportive is an important step (see Chapter 4).

Infertility tests, drugs, and surgery are expensive. Before starting your workup, discuss the projected costs of treatment and any financial problems with your physician. Basic infertility testing is also available through some women's health clinics and other private programs. They often offer reduced fees for low-income patients or those without insurance coverage. (See Chapter 3 for a discussion of the economics of infertility.)

Emotional Stress of Testing

► *The emotional stress of medical procedures has immobilized me for periods of time. My career and educational goals were often interrupted during years of tests that were expensive and time-consuming; that required specific timing and sometimes had to be repeated; that were often painful, inconclusive, and embarrassing; and that sometimes required surgery. On many occasions I would put myself and my husband through emotions I didn't realize I was capable of as a result of tests.*

Once a couple decides to have a baby, it is a bitter disappointment when menstruation occurs each month. After years of careful contraception, it is maddening to find conception difficult or even unattainable. Anxiety, marital stress, anger, and loss of self-esteem are all common reactions. It is critical to address these emotions, as well as your medical

TABLE 8.1 Female Infertility Workup Tests

Procedure	Purpose	Benefits, Risks, and Inconveniences	Approximate Cost (1987)*
Initial Visit—interview, physical exam, routine lab work, semen analysis for male partner	To gather medical history of both partners, detect obvious anatomical or physical abnormalities which may be impairing fertility	May reveal causes of infertility without necessity of more costly, invasive testing	About $125 plus any lab work ordered
Basal Body Temperature (BBT) Chart	To determine length of cycles, and based on temperature elevation, probable ovulation date	Becomes tedious and stressful, affecting couple's sex life	Cost of good, reliable thermometer
Post Coital Test (PCT or Sims-Huhner)	To observe the quality and cellular characteristics of mid-cycle cervical mucus and the sperm's reaction to it	Couple is pressured to have intercourse two to four hours before the office visit; pelvic exam necessary to obtain mucus sample	$40–50
Hysterosalpingogram (HSG)	To diagnose tubal blockages, and in some cases, uterine abnormalities	Injection of dye may clear tubes; requires clamping of uterus which may cause cramps or discomfort; small risk of infection	$185 for radiologist and hospital charges
Serum Progesterone, FSH, LH, Prolactin	To measure level of various hormones during the menstrual cycle	Simple, non-invasive blood tests which may indicate reasons for infertility	$46 to $60, depending on the test
Endometrial Biopsy	To examine endometrial cells for luteal phase characteristics—a good indication whether ovulation is occuring	Can cause painful cramping—many specialists use mini para-cervical block	About $155 for both physician's and laboratory charges
Laparoscopy	To view the exterior surfaces of the reproductive organs and abdomen; only reliable way to diagnose some pelvic problems, e.g. endometriosis and external tubal adhesions	Requires hospitalization (usually outpatient); stresses and risks of anesthesia and surgery	About $2500 for surgeon's and hospital charges

* Costs may vary in different geographic areas. These charges are based on an average of the fees of several San Francisco area hospitals, specialists, and laboratories.

problems, during this time. By entering the workup process with an informed and positive attitude, couples can optimize their chances of success, feel some degree of control over their treatment, and enhance their love and respect for each other.

The Initial Infertility Visit

► *I went to that first visit feeling vulnerable and scared. I was relieved that before the physical exam we met with our specialist in his private office. He and his staff were friendly, and I felt good about seeking answers and help for my problem. But I also felt angry that I had to go through this at all.*

It is recommended that both partners attend the first visit to meet the specialist, discuss their medical histories and personal concerns, and help plan the course of their workup.

The initial visit begins in the specialist's private office. The doctor will take a medical history, which includes the age of each partner, any medical problems, past contraception methods, marital history, present relationship, previous pregnancies by past or present partner and the outcome, past surgeries, and the duration of infertility.

Next the woman is shown to an examining room and asked to undress. She is given either a large single paper drape or two coverings for her breasts and pelvic area. The physician will perform a complete physical examination, checking the thyroid gland, breasts, pelvis, heart, lungs, and abdomen. This examination will determine whether she is in good health and without obvious gynecological abnormalities.

A PAP smear is usually done, and routine blood tests and urinalysis may be ordered. If excessive body hair or other indications of hormonal imbalance are noted, appropriate blood tests may be ordered.

Some specialists also introduce the BBT chart at this time. The couple may be asked to record daily basal temperature for a few cycles. To optimize chances for pregnancy, intercourse is usually recommended every other day around the time of ovulation.

Unless the initial examination reveals a specific problem, the workup usually begins with the simple, noninvasive, and least costly tests: semen analysis, postcoital test, blood tests, and hysterosalpingogram. Pregnancy occasionally occurs during the testing period. Otherwise the workup progresses to more complex, invasive, and expensive tests: endometrial biopsy, laparoscopy, and perhaps surgery.

If time allows, many couples continue going for tests and appointments together to ask questions, discuss test results, and plan the next step of the workup.

Semen Analysis

The semen analysis, a simple procedure, should always be done at the beginning of the workup. In the past many women endured needless tests when in fact the problem was caused by male infertility. This test may be ordered by an internist or gyneclogist before the infertility specialist is consulted.

The couple is referred to a urologist if the semen analysis is abnormal. (For a complete discussion of this test and of male infertility, see Chapters 15 and 16). If the semen analysis is normal, testing should begin on the female partner.

The Basal Body Temperature (BBT) Chart

► *Those damn charts! Nothing in my story has stayed more constant than my hatred for them. But I took my temperature religiously. Maybe, just maybe, if I was a good girl, I would get pregnant.*

Chances for pregnancy are greatly increased by timing intercourse around ovulation. The BBT chart is a graph the patient uses to plot daily basal temperature during the menstrual cycle. It is an indirect measure of ovulation based on progesterone secretion. The woman's temperature must be taken daily upon awakening and prior to *any* activity. A standard oral thermometer may be used, although BBT thermometers with minute gradations are also sold.

A textbook-perfect graph will show a low baseline temperature during and after menstruation. Prior to ovulation there will be a drop in temperature, followed by a sharp rise after an ovum is released. The rise, caused by a release of progesterone, indicates an ovum is ready for fertilization providing other factors are also favorable. If pregnancy occurs, the basal temperature will remain elevated. Otherwise, decreased hormonal secretions trigger menstruation and the temperature falls to basal level again.

Are BBT Charts Necessary?

For many infertile couples the BBT chart is a source of stress and anxiety. Sex becomes scheduled, with a resulting loss of spontaneity, and disappointment increases each month that menstruation occurs. Too often couples live by the chart and find themselves only making love around their "fertile time," a pattern that can undermine even the most stable relationship.

BASAL BODY TEMPERATURE CHART. Note that in the first graph there was no chance for conception because intercourse did not occur at the time of ovulation. During the next cycle the timing was better and pregnancy followed.

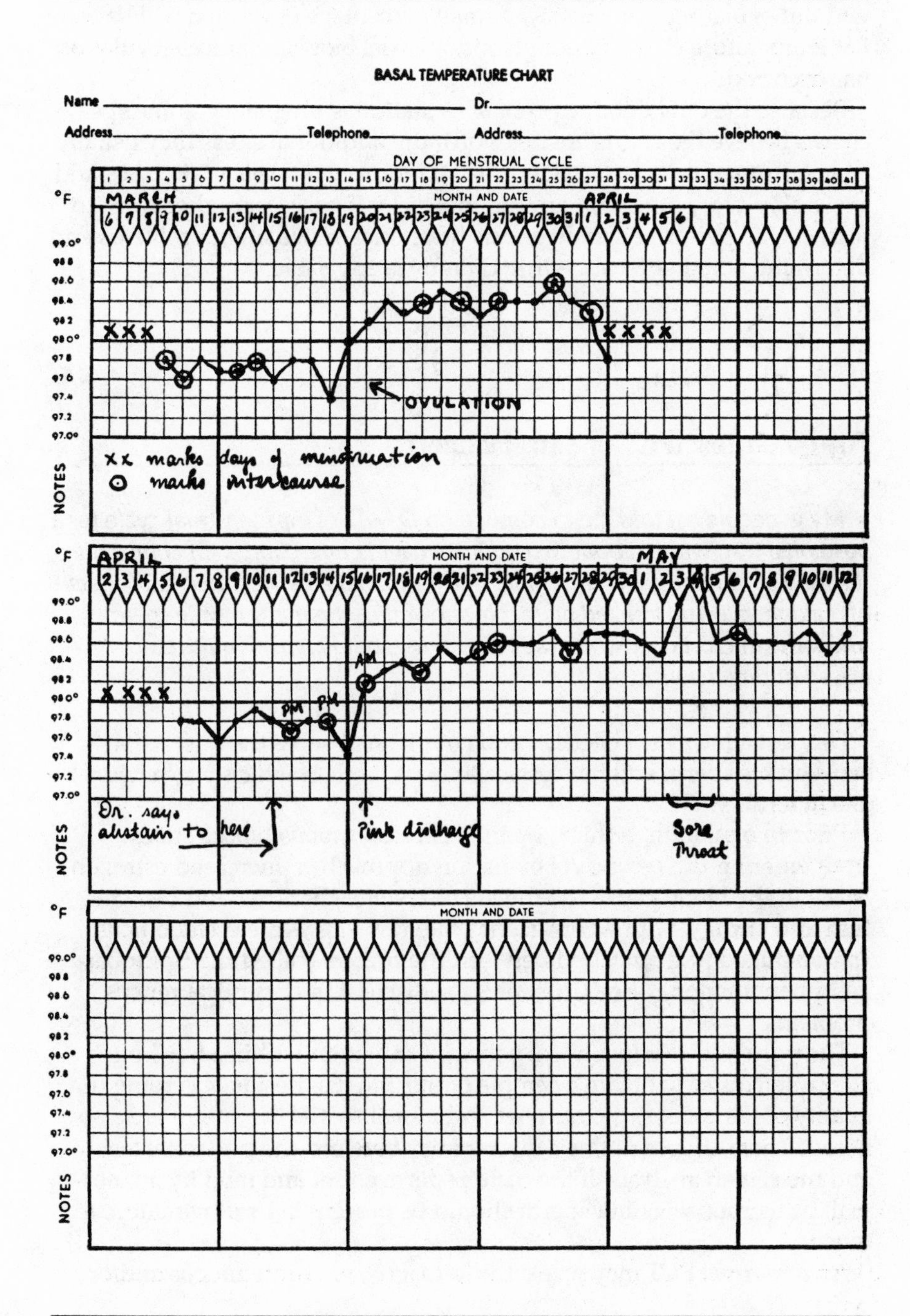

There is much controversy among specialists about the accuracy of BBT charts. Many women do not experience sharply defined drops or rises in their cycles. In rare cases the ovaries will secrete progesterone without ovulating. Conversely, a small percentage of women will have flat temperature charts although endometrial biopsies indicate ovulation has occurred.

Because the only definite proof of ovulation is pregnancy, some specialists believe the charts are not worth the additional stress they usually create. Instead they recommend sexual intimacy *throughout the cycle,* and preferably every other day around midcycle. If necessary other workup tests can be performed to diagnosis hormonal or ovulation problems and determine whether fertility drug therapy is advisable.

Postcoital Test (PCT or Sims-Hühner)

► *My gynecologist told me to come in on Day 12 of my menstrual cycle for a postcoital test, within about two hours of having intercourse. Of course the doctor was very busy that morning. But we managed a very mechanical act of making love and trekked on in. He showed us the many motile sperm under the microscope, which was reassuring; but I also felt quite embarrassed during the visit.*

This test allows the specialist and couple to observe the interaction between his sperm and her cervical mucus, both of which play a critical role in fertility.

Prior to ovulation, a thick, opaque cervical mucus blocks sperm from entering the cervix. As ovulation approaches, increased estrogen levels in the blood cause the mucus to change character and become thin and stringy, with a consistency like raw egg whites. The mucus can be pulled and stretched between the fingers (called the Spinnbarkeit phenomenon). (See Chapter 9 for discussion of cervical mucus problems.)

The postcoital test involves a pelvic examination within a few hours after intercourse to obtain a sample of this mucus. Beside observing the quality of the mucus, the number and movement of the sperm are also noted. There should not be a discrepancy between the postcoital test and the semen analysis. If the male's sperm count and motility are normal, numerous wiggling sperm should be present in healthy midcycle mucus.

An abnormal PCT may reveal thick, cloudy, or scanty mucus and/or few or no living sperm. The pH and acidity level of the mucus, which affect receptivity to sperm, can also be measured. An improper chemical balance or sperm antibodies within the mucus may be among the factors responsible for an abnormal test.

Though painless, the test is likely to involve some inconvenience as it cannot easily be scheduled in advance. Some patients find it embarrassing as well. Because pH and acidity factors can change within several hours, couples are usually advised to have intercourse two to four hours before the office visit. If such timing is difficult for you, and repeated postcoital tests are necessary, discuss your concerns with your specialist.

Hysterosalpingogram (HSG)

► *I was very anxious as I awaited my HSG, terrified that it would reveal blocked tubes. Since I'd had an IUD and probably some mild pelvic infections, I suspected that the tubes were the source of my infertility. The procedure was painful but quick. To my joy, my body told me that my tubes were open as I felt the dye pass through them. Simultaneously I saw it all on the screen as my gynecologist and the radiologist also watched. The results were so positive that I didn't mind the physical pain. Even as it occurred, I imagined I would perceive the pain of childbirth.*

This X-ray study can diagnose tubal blockage or uterine abnormalities. Many specialists like to attend the test to supervise the procedure and observe the results.

The patient lies on the examining table with her legs elevated in stirrups. To control the motion of the uterus, the physician or radiologist places a clamp on the cervix, which often produces unpleasant or painful cramping. A radiopaque dye is then injected into the uterus. As the dye moves through the pelvic organs, an X-ray machine photographs the revealed outline. If the Fallopian tubes are open, the dye spills out the ends and is absorbed by the body. There can be a therapeutic benefit to the procedure as the flushing of the tubes can improve their functioning. Some women become pregnant within three to six months following the test, despite long periods of prior infertility. On the other hand, the introduction of a foreign substance into the sterile body cavity does create a slight risk of infection. A preventive treatment of oral antibiotics is sometimes prescribed before the procedure and continued for several days afterward.

An HSG will not reveal adhesions on the exterior of the tubes or microscopic damage to the tubal lining resulting from a previous infection. (See the Laparoscopy section below and Chapter 11 for further discussion of these problems.)

Serum Progesterone Test and the Endometrial Biopsy

► *My specialist smiled and said, "Your progesterone level is sky high!" This made me feel good. I tried to concentrate on this part of my fertility, which was healthy and normal.*

► *I always administer a mini paracervical block to my patient before performing an endometrial biopsy. Without a mild anesthetic, this test can be unnecessarily painful and uncomfortable.*

These two tests investigate whether ovulation is occurring and the uterine (endometrial) lining is being adequately prepared to nourish a fertilized egg. A simple blood test, taken around Day 21 of the cycle, measures the level of progesterone hormone. An elevated level would suggest that ovulation has occurred.

Different types of endometrial tissue form during the cycle depending on the amounts of estrogen and progesterone in the blood. Progesterone-formed tissue, usually present after ovulation, is necessary to sustain pregnancy. Later in the workup an endometrial biopsy may be performed to check whether the endometrial tissue has properly responded to the elevated progesterone level.

The biopsy is usually done close to menstruation, preferably Day 27. Couples who worry about affecting an early pregnancy prefer to use contraception during this cycle. Because this test causes some discomfort and pain, most specialists administer a mini paracervical block before the biopsy is performed.

The patient is prepared for a pelvic examination. After explaining the procedure, the specialist inserts a small curette (a spoonlike instrument) through the cervical canal and retrieves a bit of uterine lining. Some specialists prefer to use tubing attached to a mild suction device, a quick and painless process.

The tissue is examined microscopically. It should resemble postovulatory cells in character and hormonal content. The results of the serum progesterone, endometrial biopsy, and postcoital tests can indicate whether a problem exists within the uterus, or the ovaries are not producing the hormones necessary to establish a favorable endometrium.

A fertilized ovum may be unable to implant in a poorly developed endometrial lining, and early spontaneous abortion can occur without the woman ever being aware of a pregnancy. A progesterone deficiency, which may be exacerbated by poor general health and nutrition, can sometimes be treated with hormones.

Rubins Test (Tubal Insufflation)

This procedure, in which carbon dioxide gas is passed through the tubes under pressure, was once used extensively to check if the Fallopian tubes were open. It has now been replaced by the hysterosalpingogram. The Rubins test can be painful, will verify only that *one* tube is open, and does not reveal tubal blockages or uterine irregularities. Most infertility specialists consider this test unnecessary and outdated.

Hormonal Blood Tests

There are many hormones involved in the functioning of the menstrual cycle. If the endometrial biopsy, postcoital tests, and HSG do not reveal a cause for continued infertility, the specialist may suggest hormonal testing as the next step. Serum (blood) tests can check the levels of estrogen, FSH, LH, prolactin, and other specific hormones in the bloodstream during various phases of the menstrual cycle.

In rare cases the test results indicate the need for further investigation of the patient's pituitary, thyroid, or adrenal glands. Referral may be made to an endocrinologist, or the specialist may recommend further blood work or a CAT scan X-ray of the pituitary gland (see Chapter 9).

Laparoscopy

► *I was afraid of the laparoscopy both because it was surgery and because of what it might reveal. I both wanted a reason for why I was infertile and dreaded knowing it. I did, however, have a great deal of confidence in my specialist. Before we went to the hospital, my husband and I took a long walk on the beach. Then we checked into the same day surgery unit. The nurses were friendly and supportive, and the anesthesiologist spoke with me beforehand. As I went into surgery, I felt a great sense of relief. At last I would know something, and this awful uncertainty would be over.*

Laparoscopy, which permits the surgeon to view the exterior surfaces of the reproductive organs and abdomen, is usually performed at the end of the workup. It can be a useful diagnostic tool when other tests have not revealed a cause for continued infertility. Like all surgical procedures, laparoscopy poses a small risk of adverse reactions to anesthesia or abdominal damage from the procedure itself. It is also expensive (in 1987 surgeon and hospital bills totaled about $2500) and is usually performed under general anesthesia.

The procedure is usually quick, uncomplicated, and done on an outpatient basis. You'll be notified about preop examinations, preliminary lab work, and admission procedures. Most hospitals have a special care unit, usually called Same Day Surgery, where you'll report several hours before the procedure. After you sign consent forms, you'll be given a locker for your clothing, and a hospital gown and paper coverings for your head and feet. Your mate or a friend can usually wait with you until an operating room is available. Before you enter surgery, an anesthesiologist will discuss risks and complications with you.

During the surgery, a laparoscope (which resembles a thin telescope

THE LAPAROSCOPY

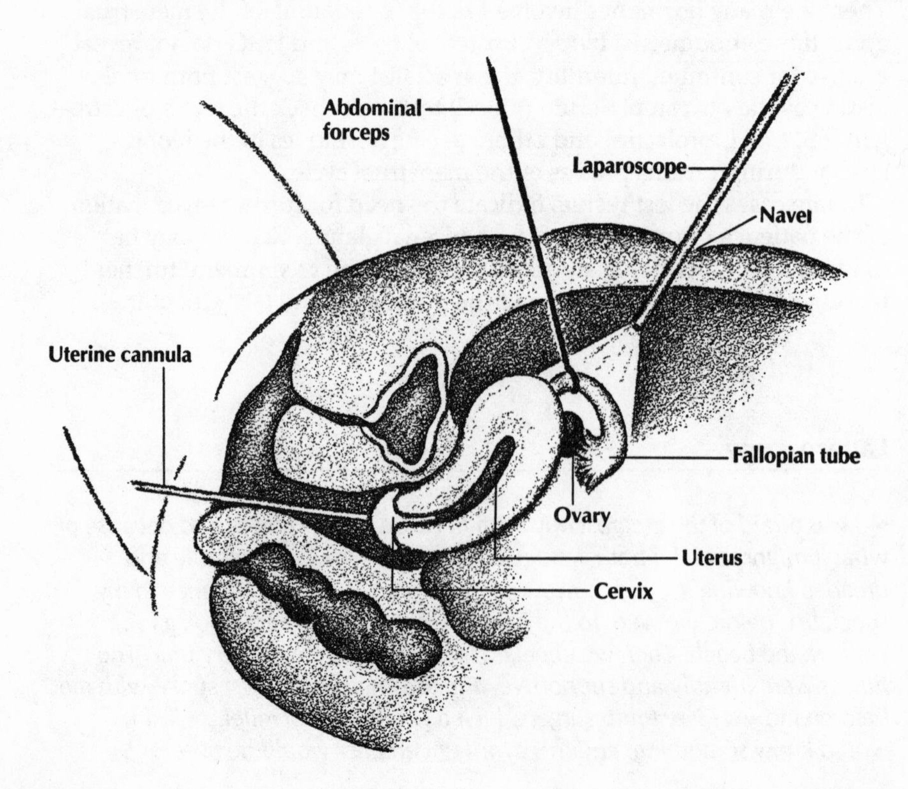

with a light at the end) is inserted through a small incision in the navel. Minor surgery can also be performed at this time. For example, adhesions can be cut (or burned by laser) through the small laparoscopic incision, freeing the tube to perform its function of transporting the egg to the uterus. Some women become pregnant after removal of tubal adhesions during laparoscopy.

After surgery you are taken to Recovery to regain partial consciousness and then back to Same Day Surgery until you're ready for discharge. Your specialist will probably review the laparoscopy with either you or your mate and leave instructions for postop care and activity. The "bandaid" incision across your navel will heal quickly. Most women require two to three days to recover, during which they feel tenderness in the abdomen and a sore throat from the anesthesia. Analgesics may be prescribed for cramps and gas discomfort.

Laparoscopy and other outpatient surgery can raise intense feelings. See Chapter 5 for a detailed discussion of the physical and emotional dynamics of surgery.

Coping with the Stress of the Infertility Workup

► *When my HSG revealed open tubes, we decided to spend a day rejoicing. I'd put off having the HSG for months, not wanting to know if the results were disappointing. We took a ride along the coast and had a marvelous dinner at a restaurant that had been highly recommended.*

In addition to those offered in other chapters, the following suggestions may be helpful during your workup:

- Educate yourself about the workup tests. Learn all you can about your tests and any problems that are diagnosed. Acquiring knowledge and information will give you a sense of control. Ask your physician for references. Some RESOLVE chapters and the national office also offer printouts about the workup tests and various medical problems.
- Work together with your specialist. Take an active role in planning the course of treatment, and call your doctor when you have questions, concerns, or need more information. If you are sensitive to pain or discomfort, ask about the use of analgesia or local anesthesia.
- Be prepared for unfavorable test results. Some of your tests may reveal a problem. This is shocking, frightening, and disappointing news. Allow yourself time to feel and absorb these emotions. One woman gave herself 24 hours to "hit bottom and lick my wounds" before fac-

ing any more. Negative test results may also reveal a reason for your infertility, perhaps a problem that can be treated. In this sense they open the door for action.

- Celebrate positive test results. A positive test result indicates one area where your body is healthy and functioning properly. Take pride in this sign of your body's strength and well-being. Share your happiness with your mate, perhaps with a romantic dinner or special outing. If a test result is unexpectedly positive, celebrate in a *big* way; let your imagination run wild!

CHAPTER 9

Hormonal Problems and Their Treatment

► *I had always thought of ovulation as such a simple task. But when I started charting those temperature graphs, I realized how irregularly I ovulated. It saddened me to think my body was having such a difficult time releasing an egg, and I dreaded taking drugs to help it happen.*

The coordinated secretion of hormones that culminates in the maturation and release of a fertile egg is staggeringly complex, requiring an intricate sequence of interactions between the hypothalamus, pituitary, and ovaries. This miraculous process is described more fully in "Human Reproduction."

Unfortunately the slightest disruption can affect the delicate chemical balances necessary for ovulation to occur. In fact between 2 and 3 percent of *all* women of reproductive age suffer from secondary amenorrhea (an absence of three or more consecutive menstrual cycles after puberty). Many other women ovulate irregularly. In all, between 20 and 30 percent of female infertility patients experience ovulatory problems.

Other women suffer from inadequate hormone production during the third, or luteal, phase of their cycles. This imbalance can cause problems with implantation or early gestation of a fertilized embryo. Hormonal imbalances can also affect the production and consistency of cervical mucus so that some or all of the sperm may not be able to penetrate the mucus and enter the uterus, thus preventing or impairing the chances for fertilization.

Factors That Can Disrupt Ovulation

In most cases it is not known why a woman ovulates irregularly or suffers from secondary amenorrhea. A thorough infertility workup does not reveal any organic problem in these women. After a reasonable investigation of physical and hormonal factors, the specialist may recommend drug treatment to induce ovulation. Other women have problems involving the ovaries, hypothalamus, and pituitary that disrupt or halt the ovulation process.

Polycystic Ovarian Disease

Polycystic ovarian disease (PCO), also called Stein-Leventhal syndrome, is caused by hormonal imbalances that disrupt the ovulation process. Named for the multiple cysts that often form on the ovaries in response to these imbalances, PCO occurs in between 1 and 4 percent of all women, and about 50 percent of those who suffer from secondary amenorrhea.

WHAT CAUSES IT? PCO is a cyclical, self-perpetuating condition. Although men and women normally have correspondingly appropriate amounts of both female and male hormones in their systems, for unknown reasons women with PCO have elevated androgen (male hormone) levels. These levels are toxic to the developing follicles within the ovary. Their growth is arrested and pea-sized cysts are formed on the surface of the ovary. These cysts, many times smaller than those ovarian cysts that require surgical removal, produce some estrogen, which slows follicle stimulating hormone (FSH) production. Although leutinizing hormone (LH) levels are slightly elevated in response to the estrogen production, ovulation does not occur because the ovarian follicles have atrophied. This results in an absence of progesterone hormone. Androgen levels remain high and the cycle repeats itself.

SYMPTOMS Symptoms include elevated androgen levels, which can be detected by a blood test. Women with PCO also have a history of very irregular or nonexistent menstrual cycles. Excessive hair growth on the face, breasts, and abdomen occurs in 70 percent of patients. Obesity and enlarged ovaries are other symptoms.

TREATMENT At one time, PCO was treated by surgically removing a wedge of the ovary. *This procedure is no longer recommended.*

If a pregnancy is desired, clomiphene is usually prescribed to induce ovulation. Otherwise oral contraceptives may be recommended to add progesterone to the cycle.

Post–Birth Control Pill Syndrome

► *I took the pill for four years. After I stopped, it was a long nine months before my periods resumed. I was afraid I wouldn't ovulate again without drug treatment.*

Birth control pills prevent ovulation by suppressing the activity of the pituitary and hypothalamus glands. After the pill is stopped, it may take from 3 to 12 months before the body resumes normal ovulatory cycles.

Most specialists prefer to let the body resume its cycles naturally. For about 5 percent of women who stop taking the pill, however, a year or more will pass without a resumption of ovulation. These are usually women who experienced irregular periods before taking the pill and are thought to have a predisposition to ovulatory problems. In these cases fertility drug treatment may be considered.

Hyperprolactinism

Prolactin, a hormone present in both men and women, is manufactured by the pituitary gland. Its production, however, is probably controlled by the hypothalamus through complex hormonal interactions. Prolactin prepares a woman's breasts for lactation during pregnancy and remains elevated while she nurses. Its other functions in both sexes are not fully understood.

Tranquilizers, some high blood pressure medications, tiny tumors, hypothyroidism, or unknown factors can cause excessive secretion of this hormone (hyperprolactinism), which occurs in about 15 percent of women with ovulatory problems. This imbalance can interfere with ovulation or implantation. Because prolactin levels are elevated as long as a woman nurses, lactation has a reputation as a natural (but unreliable) contraceptive.

SYMPTOMS About 30 percent of patients with hyperprolactinism have milk in their breasts, a condition called galactorrhea. (Breast milk is not always visible; in some cases, it may be detected by massaging the breasts and gently squeezing the nipples.) Other symptoms may include decreased vaginal secretions, irregular ovulation or amenorrhea, and luteal phase defect. Not all women with these problems, however, have elevated prolactin levels.

DIAGNOSIS Although prolactin has been recognized for a century, a simple blood test for measuring its presence was not developed until the midseventies. Specialists now consider between 0 and 20 ng/ml (ng = billionth of a gram) in the normal range. Higher levels are considered abnormal and can exceed 100 ng/ml when pituitary tumors are present.

PITUITARY TUMOR TESTING

► *My blood test revealed a high prolactin level. I had to have an X-ray of my pituitary gland done to ensure there wasn't a tumor there causing the imbalance.*

Pituitary tumor? *The very phrase wreaked such terror in me that I nearly fainted at the suggestion. I closed my eyes and tried to feel if something was there.*

Prolactin-secreting pituitary adenomas, which in all reported cases have been benign, occur in 5 percent of women with secondary amenorrhea. Although this can be a frightening prospect, it is important to remember that the pituitary gland is not part of the brain but is located below it; pituitary adenomas will not impair or affect brain function.

When a blood serum test reveals hyperprolactinism, your specialist may recommend a CAT (computerized axial tomography) scan to check for adenomas. Usually performed on an outpatient basis in the hospital, this X-ray technique produces a computerized picture of the brain and its adjacent structures with remarkable accuracy. The scan uses less radiation than a regular head X-ray and produces photographs of minute, carefully defined areas of the pituitary gland, which can reveal adenomas or cysts.

The patient must lie still on an X-ray table for 30 to 45 minutes, a difficult task if one feels anxious or nervous. The machine is kept in a cool room, so ask for a blanket if you feel uncomfortable. During the scan your head may be encompassed by the machine and this can cause sensory deprivation. Some patients are positioned with their heads resting below their shoulders in a recessed, padded area. This can also be disorienting. Let the technician know which position is most comfortable for you. Visualizing relaxing, peaceful scenes can relieve boredom and fear.

Although the films are taken by a technician, only a radiologist may interpret and discuss the results. The radiologist will consult your specialist and discuss the findings.

TREATMENT Because pituitary adenomas are benign and rarely measure more than ⅓ inch in diameter, surgery is rarely recommended; instead adenomas are usually treated with the drug bromocriptine. It is thought that this drug shrinks the tumor while the medication is taken, but it is not known whether the tumor will grow again after the drug is stopped. (Bromocriptine is described more fully below.)

EMOTIONAL SUPPORT A suspected pituitary tumor is a frightening prospect. It is important to remember, however, that most pituitary adenomas are benign and bromocriptine treatment offers encouraging success rates. For reassurance and emotional support, many RESOLVE chapters can refer you to other women and men who have been tested and treated for pituitary adenomas.

Premature Ovarian Failure

Premature ovarian failure is a condition in which the ovaries "shut down" and cease to manufacture hormones before menopause has naturally occurred. This problem occurs in about 10 percent of ovulation problems associated with infertility. Diagnosis is made by physical examination, laboratory tests, and, for women under 30 years of age, a chromosome study (karyotyping).

Premature ovarian failure can be caused by a number of factors. There may be decreased numbers of oocytes (germ cells), destruction of these cells after birth, or an acceleration of the natural disintegration process. Sometimes exposure to radiation or chemotherapy can affect the functioning of the ovaries. An autoimmune response, some types of chromosomal abnormalities, and perhaps even genetic tendency may also be underlying causes.

Premature ovarian failure is an irreversible condition. Some specialists recommend treatment with estrogen to prevent osteoporosis and atrophy of the genital tract. Although it is extremely unlikely, a pregnancy may occur after this drug treatment.

Absence of Gonadotropin-Releasing Hormone (GnRH)

Originating from the hypothalamus, GnRH triggers the release of FSH and LH from the pituitary gland. The hypothalamus may cease to secrete GnRH in response to stress or for other unknown reasons, and this may in turn halt the pituitary gland's hormonal activity.

At first, GnRH was administered to patients in continuous doses of either too great or too little quantity. It has since been discovered that the brain releases GnRH in a pulsing manner. The ovulation pump, a fairly new device that mimics the brain's method of release, is discussed in the fertility drug section below.

Luteal Phase Defects

► *Diagnosing my luteal phase problem required numerous endometrial biopsies. I also lost several early pregnancies. I felt like I was on an emotional roller coaster of hope, disappointment, and grief.*

The luteal phase of a woman's cycle is normally the 10 to 14 days between ovulation and her next menstrual period. When this half of the cycle lasts nine days or less, or inadequate levels of progesterone hormone are secreted during this phase, the patient is thought to have a luteal phase defect. This complaint, which occurs in about 5 percent of infertility patients, is a poorly understood set of hormonal fluctuations that prevent the body from achieving or sustaining pregnancy. Women with this problem may also suffer multiple miscarriages.

Luteal phase problems may be caused by a low output of progesterone hormone, which results in an inadequate maturation of the endometrial lining. The embryo then has difficulty implanting and surviving its early gestation. It is also thought that a high prolactin level or use of clomiphene may contribute to luteal phase problems.

DIAGNOSIS A luteal phase defect is usually diagnosed by a low blood serum progesterone test after ovulation (taken at about Day 21), along with an endometrial biopsy (performed around Day 27) that indicates a development lag in the maturation of the endometrium of two or more days. Known to occur sporadically in many women, luteal phase defect should be documented in at least two successive menstrual cycles before a diagnosis is made.

TREATMENT Luteal phase problems are usually treated with clomiphene, clomiphene and human chorionic gonadotropin (HCG), or natural progesterone suppositories (although the latter treatment has not yet been approved by the FDA). Forms of synthetic progesterone, such as birth control pills, are not recommended because they can cause birth defects. Some specialists recommend intramuscular injections of progesterone to support early pregnancy in women with a history of miscarriage. However, there is controversy among experts about whether this is effective.

Infertility specialists also differ on whether to use clomiphene to treat luteal phase defect problems. Paradoxically this drug sometimes causes luteal phase problems in women with normal ovulatory cycles by affecting progesterone secretion. The best treatment for luteal phase defect problems remains elusive.

EMOTIONAL IMPACT Luteal phase problems exact a heavy emotional toll. Frequent endometrial biopsies may be required, and there are often false pregnancy hopes or miscarriages. If you suffer from this problem, be sure to seek emotional support, as well as competent medical care.

Cervical Mucus Problems

The cervix contains more than a hundred tiny glands that secrete mucus throughout the menstrual cycle. This mucus, which changes character and consistency as estrogen levels shift, plays a critical role in fertility.

During most of the cycle cervical mucus is quite acidic, thick, and cloudy. It creates a barrier that prevents bacteria, sperm, and other foreign substances from entering the uterus. When sperm encounter this type of mucus, they usually die within a few hours.

In response to a complex interaction of hormonal signals estrogen levels increase as the body prepares to release an egg. Ideally, about two days before ovulation occurs the tiny cervical opening (os) dilates slightly, and the glands increase mucus production about 30-fold. The mucus, composed of about 98 percent water with traces of salts and proteins, becomes thin and clear. The pH of the mucus becomes slightly alkaline, a "sperm-friendly" solution that serves as a buffer to the vagina's normally acidic environment.

Under the microscope this ideal mucus has a fernlike appearance. Its cells actually form long narrow filaments with large open spaces between them. Over the course of several days the sperm swim through these spaces, enter the uterus, and eventually move through the Fallopian tubes in search of an ovum. For up to three days the mucus acts as a reservoir for continuous release of sperm into the uterus. After ovulation occurs, estrogen levels decrease. In response the cervical mucus becomes thick and opaque and again forms a barrier.

It is important to note, however, that each woman's body varies in the amount and consistency of midcycle mucus. Some women easily detect mucus in the vagina or on toilet tissue. Some can actually pull and stretch it between their fingers. Other women may feel "dry" in the vagina when in fact perfect midcycle mucus is present near the cervix.

Some women also get pregnant with scanty or thick mucus. Inadequate or scant midcycle mucus, however, may impair fertility in some cases. It is estimated that 10 to 15 percent of female infertility patients have a mucus problem, although it is difficult to determine whether this is the *sole* factor in the couple's infertility. In many cases the cause of mucus problems is not known, although hormonal abnormalities are often a contributing factor.

The Hühner (or postcoital) test, performed during the female infertility workup, checks the quality and quantity of midcycle mucus and the sperm's reaction to it. "Poor" midcycle cervical mucus is usually thick and cellular and may contain white or red blood cells.

TREATMENT There are, unfortunately, few effective treatments for cervical mucus problems. Some infertility specialists prescribe estrogen pills for seven to ten days prior to ovulation to stimulate mucus production. Artificial insemination by husband's sperm (AIH) may also be recommended. The semen may be placed directly into the uterus, bypassing the mucus completely. Intrauterine insemination offers a 25 to 30 percent success rate.

Some specialists also recommend doses of a decongestant cough syrup during the first two weeks of the cycle to increase mucus production throughout the body. Although not scientifically documented, some women report an increase in quality and quantity of cervical mucus afterward, and a few pregnancies have occurred. It is not harmful or expensive and may be worth a try if no other fertility problem has been diagnosed.

Fertility, or Ovulation-Inducing, Drugs

Four different drugs have been developed to help women who ovulate either infrequently or not at all. These drugs—clomiphene, bromocriptine, human menopausal gonadotropin, and gonadotropin-releasing hormone—are appropriate only in specific situations. Before beginning treatment with any drug, each infertile woman must be individually evaluated by her specialist. What will help one woman may not be beneficial for another.

Although the FDA has tested, and in some cases approved, the use of these drugs for fertility problems, it is important to remember that no drug is completely safe or innocuous. The long-term effects of these drugs on the patient, as well as her or his unborn children, is not known. Educate yourself about the history, side effects, and success rates of any recommended drug. Discuss any questions and concerns with your specialist, pharmacist, and others who have taken the drug. Other sources of information about fertility drugs include literature from pharmaceutical companies, the *Essential Guide to Prescription Drugs*, the *Physician's Desk Reference* (PDR), and medical libraries. (Chapter 4 includes suggestions for doing your own medical research.)

Clomiphene (brand names Serophene, Clomid)

► *Clomiphene greatly affected my moods and ability to cope. I felt these changes a day after I began the pills until about 36 hours after I stopped. I began to dread "clomiphene days," but was afraid that if I stopped taking it I wouldn't ovulate. Luckily I had no problem with ovarian cysts.*

► *I conceived my son after one cycle of clomiphene. I just couldn't ovulate without it. I was lucky it worked so quickly and I felt no ill effects.*

Clomiphene, the most commonly prescribed fertility drug, is used primarily by women who ovulate either irregularly or not at all. Clomiphene may also be prescribed to improve progesterone production after ovulation, a common cause of luteal phase defect. It is also sometimes tried to improve low sperm counts (see Chapter 15).

Hundreds of thousands of patients have taken clomiphene. It works best in patients who ovulate occasionally. It *does not* improve fertility in women with regular menstrual cycles. Clomiphene is considered a well-established, "safe" drug by the medical profession to the extent that it is not inherently dangerous or life-threatening.

An antiestrogen, clomiphene induces ovulation by tricking the pituitary into producing FSH and smaller amounts of LH. These hormones stimulate the ovary to ripen several follicles, which increases estrogen levels. When clomiphene is stopped, the hypothalamus detects the estrogen and prompts the pituitary to release a surge of LH, which stimulates ovulation.

CONTRAINDICATIONS Clomiphene should not be prescribed if large fibroid tumors are present, as it can cause them to grow. (Treatment in cases of small fibroids should be carefully discussed with your specialist.) This drug is also not appropriate for patients with ovarian cysts or liver problems.

TABLE 9.1 "Fertility" (Ovulation-Inducing) Drugs

Drug	Function	Contraindications
Clomiphene (Brand names Clomid, Serophene)	Induces ovulation by chemically stimulating the pituitary gland to produce hormones which trigger the ovulation process	May not be appropriate for patients with large fibroid tumors, ovarian cysts or liver problems
Bromocriptine (Brand name Parlodel)	Reduces pituitary's production of prolactin hormone while it is taken	May not be appropriate for patients with pituitary tumors larger than 1 cm
Human Menopausal Gonadotropin or HMG (Brand name Pergonal)	Stimulates ovary to develop follicles. In addition, an injection of Human Chorionic Gonadotropin required to trigger ovulation	May not be appropriate in cases of pituitary tumor, ovarian cysts, or ovarian or adrenal problems
Gonadotropin Releasing Hormone (GnRH)	Triggers normal pituitary hormonal activity so ovulation can occur	Because it is a natural hormone, no obvious contraindications

NOTE: This table should be read across pp. 126 and 127.

PERIODIC PELVIC EXAMINATIONS Normally clomiphene causes some ovarian enlargement, which is usually not harmful or dangerous. Ideally a follicular cyst about an inch in diameter develops, forms a corpus luteum, and dissolves if pregnancy does not occur. Although the risk of forming other types of cysts is very low if successful ovulation takes place, a woman taking clomiphene should have periodic pelvic examinations to ensure that her ovaries are not enlarging abnormally. Your specialist will advise you on how often to schedule appointments.

DOSAGE Clomiphene is administered orally, usually in doses of 50 mg daily for five days, beginning with the second to fifth day of the menstrual cycle. The dosage may be increased to as much as 250 mg per day for five to eight days if the patient does not respond.

SIDE EFFECTS Clomiphene increases estrogen in the body to higher levels than in a normal ovulatory cycle, which causes some side effects in many, but not all, women who take it. Some of these same problems also occur with birth control pills, another type of hormonal therapy. The intensity and frequency of side effects vary with each patient.

Dosage	Side Effects	1987 Cost/Cycle
Usually 50 mg/day for 5 days; dosage may be increased to 250 mg/day for 5–8 days if necessary	Vary in frequency and intensity with each patient; may include nausea, vomiting, visual problems, headache, insomnia, hot flashes, breast tenderness, heightened emotional sensitivity	$20–25
2.5 mg 2 or 3 times/day	May include nausea, nasal stuffiness, dizziness, low blood pressure, headache	About $70
Controlled doses given by injection for 9–12 days	20–40 percent possibility of multiple births; small risk of hyperstimulation syndrome; involves a great deal of emotional stress	About $1000–1500
An ovulation pump administers minute, pulsating injections every 90 minutes	No known physical side effects; patient must carry pump and attached IV tubing for one or two weeks or until ovulation occurs	About $1000 for pump plus $300/cycle for hormone, tubing, and office visits

Reported side effects include nausea, vomiting, vision problems, headache, insomnia, hot flashes, irritability, and breast tenderness. Because clomiphene can also cause dizziness or vision problems, be cautious while driving or performing chores requiring alertness. Immediately report any side effect to your specialist.

CERVICAL MUCUS CHANGES Because it is an antiestrogen, clomiphene may also diminish the quality and quantity of cervical mucus. If this happens, synthetic estrogen (Estrace or Premarin) may be prescribed from Day 8 through Day 16 of the cycle. It can be difficult to balance the clomiphene and estrogen, and dosages may need to be adjusted.

EMOTIONAL EFFECTS OF CLOMIPHENE Many women complain of intense mood swings and heightened emotional sensitivity while taking clomiphene. Besides causing personal frustration these reactions may contribute to marital stress. In addition, some physicians discount their patients' complaints about the emotional effects of clomiphene, which may cause friction between doctor and patient.

SUCCESS RATE About 80 percent of patients ovulate and about 40 percent become pregnant with clomiphene. Most pregnancies occur within the first three months of treatment, and there is a 5 to 10 percent chance of conceiving twins with clomiphene use. The 20 percent miscarriage rate associated with this drug is actually a little lower than that of the general population. It is thought that the increased progesterone levels generated by clomiphene may actually help sustain early pregnancy.

COST Clomiphene is the least expensive fertility drug. A one-cycle supply of five 50 mg tablets may range from $20 to $25 or more. It pays to shop around before ordering the drug.

Bromocriptine (brand name Parlodel)

► *I conceived my daughter after taking bromocriptine for nine cycles. Luckily I felt no side effects from it. We stopped the drug immediately after a positive early pregnancy test. Still, my baby was exposed to the drug for several weeks and I do worry about that.*

► *The initial effects were literally staggering. For two days I couldn't stand up without having the room spin. I was ready to give up when, on the the third morning, I got out of bed and, to my surprise, life was back to normal.*

Bromocriptine, a drug first marketed in 1978, controls hyperprolactinism by suppressing hypothalamic activity. *This drug does not cure hyperprolactinism,* but it will reduce prolactin levels *while it is taken*. Previous symptoms often recur when the drug is stopped. At this writing, bromocriptine has not been approved by the FDA for ovulation induction, so your informed consent is required before it can be prescribed for fertility treatment.

Before recommending treatment with this drug, your specialist may recommend a CAT scan to insure that pituitary tumors (adenomas) are not causing the imbalance. Although this medication can be used by patients with adenomas smaller than 1 cm, patients with larger tumors may not respond as well to the drug.

DOSAGE Bromocriptine is introduced slowly, usually beginning with one dose per day for a week. This gradual increase usually prevents sudden drops in blood pressure. Eventually, a dosage of 2.5 mg of the drug is taken two or three times daily with meals to alleviate nausea. The drug should be discontinued when a pregnancy is confirmed.

SIDE EFFECTS Initially many patients taking bromocriptine experience nausea, nasal stuffiness, dizziness, low blood pressure, or headache.

These symptoms usually abate with time, often after the first few doses. While your body adjusts to the drug, it is wise to avoid sudden changes in posture and to use caution when driving or engaging in activities requiring alertness.

This drug has been used extensively in Europe, Japan, and the United States for almost a decade. Its use has not been associated with a greater incidence of birth defects or miscarriage than occurs in the general population.

SUCCESS RATES About 90 percent of women will ovulate with bromocriptine as long as it is taken. Pregnancy rates range between 65 and 85 percent.

COST Each tablet costs about 75 cents. They must be taken continuously, two to three times daily—an expense of about $70 per month.

Human Menopausal Gonadotropin (HMG) (brand name Pergonal)

► *I'm now trying HMG for the fourth and last time. I've been lucky not to have any physical discomfort or side effects. Still, so much rides on each attempt—physically, financially, and emotionally.*

Yet this experience has also brought my husband and me closer. He has been trained to give me some of the shots at home. He's also come for the ultrasound tests; together we've seen the developing follicles on the screen. It's been hard not to consider each follicle as a "mini pregnancy" even though they haven't been fertilized yet! At first we even gave each one a nickname, but we soon stopped that. It was so painful when I didn't get pregnant. We both feel, though, that it has been a wonder to witness the growth of an egg. The ultrasound has given us a window into a miracle.

A very expensive and laboriously prepared medication, HMG is purified FSH and LH hormone. Developed in the early 1960s, it is a natural hormone made from the urine of postmenopausal women. When the ovary detects HMG in the blood, it assumes that FSH has been released by the pituitary. In response the ovary develops numerous follicles, even though the pituitary and hypothalamus have remained dormant. Ovulation, however, cannot occur without an injection of human chorionic gonadotropin (HCG), which simulates the presence of LH.

This drug is most often prescribed to women with low estrogen levels who do not respond to clomiphene. It may also be used in cases of polycystic ovarian disease or luteal phase defects or during IVF procedures. In some cases HMG may be taken in conjunction with clomiphene. It is also sometimes prescribed for men with low sperm counts. The use of HMG can result in multiple fetuses and, in rare cases, hyperstimulation of the ovaries. For this reason, *only specialists experienced with the use of HMG should supervise the use of this drug.*

CONTRAINDICATIONS Before HMG is prescribed, the possibility of pituitary tumor should be investigated. In addition, it should not be used if thyroid or adrenal problems or ovarian cysts are present.

PROCEDURE Treatment can begin at any time. The HMG is injected intramuscularly in controlled doses, measured in ampules, for 9 to 12 days. Some specialists will train the patient or her husband to administer the shots, a way to involve both partners and reduce some of the necessary office visits.

During treatment the patient is carefully monitored for estrogen levels, ovarian enlargement, and cervical mucus changes. When the mucus indicates ovulation is near, daily pelvic examinations, ultrasound, and blood tests are performed to monitor the number and quality of developing follicles. These tests are used to adjust the dosage of HMG. If too many follicles develop, treatment may be discontinued until these ova disintegrate and then resumed again a few weeks later.

When an ultrasound reveals that the eggs are mature, an injection of 10,000 IU of HCG is given. Ovulation should occur 24 to 36 hours later.

SIDE EFFECTS Use of HMG has always carried a high rate of multiple births. Although ultrasound techniques have reduced this likelihood, twins do occur in 20 to 40 percent of cases; the incidence of triplets or other multiple births has been reduced. Most physicians will not proceed with a cycle if more than five follicles develop (unless in vitro fertilization is being attempted.) There may also be risks of miscarriage or premature delivery.

In 3 to 5 percent of HMG cycles, excessive estrogen levels lead to hyperstimulation syndrome, characterized by ovarian enlargement, abdominal swelling, and weight gain. Severe cases of hyperstimulation require immediate hospitalization and continued observation for one to three weeks until the swelling subsides.

EMOTIONAL FACTORS The HMG treatment requires intense, almost daily involvement in office visits, injections, examinations, and monitoring tests. Because the patient and her partner can watch the maturation of the follicles, many are extremely frustrated and disappointed if ovulation or pregnancy does not occur. That HMG is offered to women who do not respond to other fertility drugs, and is thus often a final course of medical treatment, intensifies this pressure.

COST Treatment with HMG is expensive. Ampules cost about $40 each, and several dozen may be used each month. On the average, HMG use runs about $1000 to $1500 per cycle. Some medical insurance carriers will cover all or part of this expense.

SUCCESS RATES More than 75 percent of women ovulate with HMG treatment. Between 20 and 80 percent of these patients will get pregnant, depending on the nature of their hormonal problems and whether other infertility factors are present. The miscarriage rate may be slightly higher than that of the general population.

Gonadotropin-Releasing Hormone (GnRH) and the Ovulation Pump

► *I consider the pump a mixed blessing. It has given me the gift to discover my body can function normally with a little help. However, inserting the needles has often been physically painful. I've also had to make a big adjustment to physically carrying the pump and tubing around for a week or two. Still, I prefer the pump and GnRH treatment, in both a physical and emotional sense, to HMG.*

A natural hormone, GnRH can be used by women who do not respond to clomiphene, but it does not seem to help women with a luteal phase defect. A pump has been developed to administer this hormone to anovulatory women. A battery-run pump about 3 inches by 4 inches, often used by diabetics to deliver measured doses of insulin, administers a minute, pulsating injection of GnRH every 90 minutes around the clock. These small intermittent doses mimic hypothalamic stimulation of the pituitary. The body then takes over and releases the other hormones necessary for a normal cycle, although an HCG injection is often given to support ovulation.

This treatment is performed on an outpatient basis and can be started at any time. The GnRH hormone is placed in a bag inside the pump. One end of a generous length of plastic tubing is attached to the pump; the other end contains a needle, which is inserted in an arm vein and securely bandaged. The site of the needle is changed every four or five days. Long-sleeved clothing can be worn over the tubing, and the pump can be carried in a pocket or worn at the waist. The pump is needed only until ovulation has occurred.

SUCCESS RATES Most patients ovulate in one to two weeks. Pregnancy rates vary, so check with each program for their success rates.

COST In 1987, the cost of the pump was about $1000. In addition, per cycle costs ran about $300 for the drug, IV tubing, and the monitoring program.

Coping with Fertility Drugs

Many of us find it difficult to separate a fertility drug's effects from the overall physical and emotional stress of infertility. If you do experience adverse reactions to any drug, notify your specialist immediately and discuss your physical and emotional reactions with your mate. It also helps to take life a day at a time, periodically reassess your goals, and employ some of the coping suggestions offered in Part One.

CHAPTER 10

Pelvic Abnormalities and Microsurgery Treatment

► *The HSG and laparoscopy showed my ovaries swollen with cysts and the Fallopian tubes tangled around them. My specialist reviewed the major surgery with us beforehand. He said he would do his best to save both ovaries and tubes, but he was very worried about the right side.*

"We're dealing with threads here," he said.

I closed my eyes and tried to control my fear of losing part of my body.

In addition to hormonal imbalances, several types of pelvic abnormalities can impair fertility. These include blockage or scarring of the Fallopian tubes and pelvic problems found in some women who were exposed prenatally to the drug, diethylstilbestrol (DES). Endometriosis, another common pelvic problem that can affect fertility, is discussed in Chapter 11.

The Fallopian Tubes

The Fallopian tubes (oviducts) were first described by an Italian anatomist, Gabriello Fallopio, in the 1500s. Connected to the uterus and lying just above the ovaries, they play a crucial role in fertility. Their job is to retrieve an ovum as it is released from the ovary, move the sperm toward it, and transport the fertilized zygote back to the uterus for implantation. They also secrete essential chemicals vital to proper ovum and sperm interaction. In rare cases an embryo will implant in the tube and begin an ectopic pregnancy. In most cases, however, the embryo is successfully transported to the uterus.

The oviduct's external appearance has been described as a smooth tube, gradually widening to a trumpet-shaped opening containing delicate, waving tentaclelike ends resembling a sea anemone in appearance and movement. The *infundibulum* is the trumpetlike end that nestles close to the ovary. Its rounded opening, where the ovum enters, has a diameter of between ¼ and ½ inch. Fringelike projections called *fimbria* catch the ovum as it is released from the ovary. Fertilization usually occurs in this part of the tube. Fimbria can be destroyed by inflammation and do not regenerate themselves.

The infundibulum tapers into the *ampulla* section, a slightly narrower passage that runs about half the length of the tube. This in turn narrows into the *isthmus,* only about ⅛ inch in diameter, which opens into the uterine cavity. Sperm are deposited in the vagina during intercourse, pass through the cervix, are transported by both their own locomotion and uterine contractions up the uterus, and enter the tube at the isthmus.

Numerous hairlike projections called *cilia* fill the lining of a healthy Fallopian tube. Interspersed among the cilia are *secretory cells,* which release a fluid that fills the tube. The ovum floats and the sperm swim in this medium. The cilia also facilitate transportation by beating in only one direction and by inducing contractions of the muscular walls of the tube.

The Fallopian tubes are especially vulnerable to infections and to diseases such as endometriosis. In response to these conditions the tubes become inflamed, summon millions of white blood cells to destroy the invading cells, and secrete a substance that forms scar tissue (adhesions). Even filmy adhesions can impair the delicate functioning of the tubes. If the infection continues unchecked, the tubes will continue to scar and eventually will close. Rather than allow an infection to spread to the abdomen (a life-threatening condition) the tubes often seal off their ends, sacrificing fertility to ensure the body's survival.

Acute and Chronic Salpingitis (Pelvic Inflammatory Disease)

Pelvic inflammatory disease (PID) is a term commonly used to describe an infection or disease of the pelvic organs. Although pelvic infections often enter through the cervix and can affect the uterus and ovaries, it is usually the tubes that suffer fertility impairment. The most delicate part of the reproductive system, they are the most seriously affected by infection.

The medical term for PID of the Fallopian tubes is *salpingitis,* and the disease may be present in either acute or chronic form. Acute salpingitis is the active stage of inflammation, usually caused by infection from either a sexually transmitted disease or use of an intrauterine device (IUD). It is often a silent and symptomless process; many women are unaware that they have an infection and do not seek treatment. Infertility specialists rarely see a case of acute salpingitis; instead they see its aftermath. Perhaps years after the original infection a woman attempts unsuccessfully to get pregnant. During an infertility workup her specialist discovers chronic salpingitis in the form of tubal blockages, scarring, "clubbed" (sealed) ends, or chronically inflamed tissue.

Due to the increasing incidence of sexually transmitted diseases and the recent use of intrauterine contraceptive devices by many women, salpingitis has become a major health problem in the 1980s. Every year this disease is diagnosed in more than a million American women; not surprisingly their fertility has also been affected. Salpingitis now accounts for about 30 percent of female infertility problems.

Causes of Salpingitis

SEXUALLY TRANSMITTED DISEASES (STDs) In addition to the well-known venereal diseases syphilis and gonorrhea, more than 20 new varieties of STDs have been identified. These microbes may be bacterial or viral and are passed by genital, oral, or anal contact. In recent years there has been an increasing incidence of STDs. If a woman or her mate has had multiple sexual partners, she has a good chance of contracting one of these diseases during her lifetime. The most common STDs are chlamydia and gonorrhea.

Chlamydia is a cross between a bacterial and a viral disease. It is often symptomless and is difficult to diagnose, although some women experience mild to severe abdominal pain or discomfort, a high- or low-grade fever, painful intercourse or menses, spotting between periods, vaginal discharge, or fatigue. Infected men sometimes complain of painful urination or pain after intercourse. Although both sexes can contract chlamydia, it seems to affect fertility most often in women. Men usually act as carriers, although their fertility can also be impaired. Chlamydia can live in the pelvic region for many years and will slowly scar the reproductive organs if left unchecked. To prevent reinfection, both partners are treated with antibiotics such as tetracycline or erythromycin for 10 to 14 days.

Gonorrhea is a bacterial disease that is usually spread through sexual contact. Symptoms in women may include cervical discharge, painful urination, abdominal pain, fever, and vomiting. Some women, however, have no symptoms in the early stages of the infection. Men may have a discharge from the penis or painful urination, although some experience no obvious symptoms. If left unchecked, gonorrhea can result in PID and other complications. Treatment is usually attempted with penicillin; some physicians use tetracycline if the patient is allergic or sensitive to the penicillin drugs.

INTRAUTERINE DEVICES IUDs were once thought to be safe and convenient contraceptives. Many physicians now regard them as potentially dangerous devices that have contributed to fertility problems in many women. It has also been suggested that the threads attached to IUDs, which pass through the cervix and into the vagina, often serve as "ladders" to the uterus for infectious bacteria and viruses. Thousands of women developed salpingitis after using an IUD.

The Dalkon Shield has received the most publicity as a dangerous IUD. It is now believed that all IUD devices can cause reproductive problems, and that IUD users roughly double their chances of developing salpingitis compared with women who do not use these contraceptives. Their use is no longer recommended.

Diagnosis of Salpingitis

Once ovulation and cervical mucus factors have been checked, the infertility specialist usually studies the condition of the Fallopian tubes. A pelvic examination may sometimes, but not always, reveal pelvic tenderness, decreased organ mobility, an irregular uterine shape, or a palpable mass suggesting salpingitis.

TESTS OF TUBAL PATENCY Several workup tests can be performed to check whether the tubes are open (patent) and free of blockages. Hysterosalpingogram (HSG), laparoscopy, and perhaps hysteroscopy can often determine whether the tubes are open.

The presence of chronic salpingitis, however, is often not discovered until laparoscopy, usually the last procedure of the standard female workup. During laparoscopy pelvic problems, such as adhesions, blockages, or endometriosis, can be assessed before major surgery is recommended. This is a prudent approach as pregnancy rates are highest with the initial microsurgery and decline with subsequent attempts. Depending on the extent of tubal damage, in vitro fertilization (IVF) may also be a viable option.

Microsurgery Treatment for Tubal Abnormalities

► *The surgery removed my right ovary and repaired my left tube from an ectopic pregnancy. Moderate endometriosis was also found. As I came out of the anesthetic and heard this, I thought, "How will I get pregnant now?"*

Once the tube or its lining is irrevocably damaged, it cannot be replaced, restored, or regenerated. Attempts at tubal transplants have not been successful to date. There are, however, many cases where tubal blockages can be bypassed or removed with surgery in an attempt to restore fertility.

The technique of surgery by microscope, or microsurgery, was first used about 60 years ago. It was adapted for gynecological procedures in the late 1970s, and is now widely used for fertility surgery. Previously such surgery was performed without a microscope ("macrosurgery") and was not very successful in terms of subsequent pregnancies. The advent of microsurgery provided greater magnification of the tissues and finer, more delicate cutting and suturing. The needles and suturing material used are significantly smaller than those used in macrosurgery. In addition, equipment and techniques are being constantly improved and refined in this surgical specialty.

Microsurgery can sometimes be performed during laparoscopy. In most cases, however, major surgery, which requires an abdominal incision (laparatomy), is necessary for tubal repair or extensive adhesion removal.

Surgery is an intense, traumatic experience for many patients. Chapter 5 presents a thorough discussion of the physical, emotional, and psychological dynamics of anesthesia and pelvic surgery.

Who Should Perform Microsurgery?

An infertility specialist should perform microsurgery because this technique requires intensive training and experience to master. The surgeon must carefully control bleeding, precisely cut and suture diseased areas, and handle this delicate tissue gently to minimize new adhesion formation. Microsurgical techniques are costly to learn, and continuing education is necessary to keep up with technological advances. A specialist should handle one to two cases per week to keep in practice. Some sources of referral are your gynecologist, RESOLVE, or women's health clinics.

When Is Microsurgery Indicated?

Microsurgery may be recommended to remove blockages from the tubes or adhesions from the reproductive organs. It is also performed to reverse sterilization and to remove endometriosis.

A blockage can occur anywhere in the tube. Pelvic inflammatory disease or use of an IUD, for example, can form adhesions and leave the ends of the tube blocked and swollen. During surgery adhesions are carefully cut away with scissors, electrosurgical needles, or a laser. Because of the greater magnification, less tissue is damaged by cutting and suturing.

Disadvantages

Because it is so precise and meticulous, microsurgery requires more time than macrosurgery, often three hours or more. Many specialists, however, are reporting shorter microsurgery times for many procedures. Still most patients undergo general anesthesia and are subject to its attendant risks.

Microsurgery is an expensive procedure as specialized equipment and highly trained personnel are needed. In 1987 a four-hour microsurgery and a five-day hospital stay ran about $10,000. Coverage for infertility surgery varies among insurance carriers (see Chapter 3.)

Major Surgery Following Laparoscopy

The patient, her mate, and their specialist can decide whether major surgery will be done immediately after laparoscopy or at a later date. Some women and physicians prefer to discuss the findings of the laparoscopy and then schedule major surgery at a later time. Others will want surgery to proceed immediately after the laparoscopy without the patient regaining consciousness. Some surgeons also have preferences on how to schedule major surgery.

Use of Electrosurgery and Laser Surgery

Electrosurgery is a technique in which an electrical current is used to cut or remove tissue. With laser surgery, a CO_2 laser (a special sort of light beam) is used to cut or burn away (vaporize) unwanted scar tissue. Both electrosurgery and laser surgery are usually used in conjunction with other microsurgery techniques to make incisions or remove mild to moderate adhesions either during laparoscopy or major surgery.

The laser, despite its media attention, is not a magic cure-all. It is simply an accurate way to cut or destroy abnormal tissue. By setting the energy level of the machine, the surgeon can make a fine cut that also coagulates the tissue. The laser is sometimes used by itself during laparoscopy to remove filmy tubal adhesions. Although the speed of laser surgery may diminish some of the risks of anesthesia, there is controversy among specialists whether the use of a laser results in less subsequent adhesion formation. At this time laser surgery does not offer better pregnancy rates than electrosurgery. However, more hospitals are acquiring laser equipment, and the medical community is carefully assessing the success rates and advantages of this technique for fertility treatment. RESOLVE maintains current information and an updated list of centers offering this option.

Risk of Ectopic Pregnancy After Tubal Microsurgery

The pregnancy rate in women having tubal surgery to correct problems caused by infection is fairly low (10 to 50 percent at best), and the odds that an ectopic pregnancy will occur are five to ten times greater for these women than for those in the general population. Depending on the overall condition of the tube, there is also a risk of ectopic pregnancy if the fimbria are absent.

Adhesion Formation Following Surgery

After surgery the body sometimes forms adhesions during the healing process. In most cases this does not create a problem. It is, however, an unfortunate occurrence in terms of fertility surgery. Scar tissue formed after such surgery may contribute to continued fertility problems.

In an attempt to inhibit scarring some specialists prescribe steroids, antibiotics, and other drugs, which are administered intravenously immediately after surgery. Other specialists place special solutions, such as dextran, in the abdominal cavity during surgery to discourage adhesion formation. Still there is a 30 percent chance that adhesions will form and again impair tubal function. This scarring usually occurs within the first few weeks after surgery, and there is no way to know beforehand which patients will be affected.

Some specialists will perform a laparoscopy four to six weeks after surgery for a second look. At this time adhesion formation is fresh and can perhaps be broken up through the laparoscope. If pregnancy does not occur after 6 to 12 months, other specialists recommend a second laparoscopy to check whether scarring has again impaired tubal patency and function.

Second and Subsequent Microsurgeries

The chances for pregnancy are 5 to 25 percent (or about halved) with the second major surgery. Percentages steadily decrease with subsequent surgeries. In vitro fertilization currently offers a 10 to 20 percent chance for pregnancy, and it is hoped that these success rates will improve as IVF techniques are perfected. The couple and their specialist may consider IVF a better choice after one unsuccessful microsurgery attempt.

DES

► *The presence of so many DES-exposed people in our midst is not the only reason for concern about this issue. The DES story left us "sadder but wiser" about the dangers of drug use, especially in pregnancy, and about the fallibility of drug testing and surveillance. We may never be able to guarantee against similar errors, but the lessons of DES should inspire caution among consumers and providers alike when examining the web of risks and benefits of medical technologies.*

JOAN EMERY, MPH
DES Action USA

Diethylstilbestrol (DES) is a synethetic form of estrogen still used as a "day after" contraceptive and lactation inhibitor. For many years it was also added to poultry and livestock feeds. Between 1941 and the early 1970s, DES was prescribed to millions of pregnant women (in an estimated 10 percent of all pregnancies during this time) to prevent miscarriage. Its use during pregnancy continued for nearly two decades even though studies performed in 1953 found DES ineffective in preventing miscarriage. "DES daughters and sons" are those offspring whose mothers took diethylstilbestrol during pregnancy.

Did My Mother Take DES?

There is a wide range of known and suspected side effects associated with DES exposure. It is helpful for DES offspring to discover the dosage and length of time they were exposed prenatally. When both patient and physician have this information, early detection and careful monitoring of health-related problems is possible.

Unfortunately there are many women and men who are unaware of their prenatal exposure to DES because their mothers are not sure whether they took the drug during pregnancy. DES Action USA, a nationwide consumer advocacy group, urges anyone born between 1941 and 1972 to "ask your mother." They can provide information and suggestions for tracing medical records. (In many states patients have a legal right to information contained in their medical records.) DES Action USA has many chapters and is an excellent resource for emotional support, information, and medical referrals (see Appendix A).

Effects on Health and Fertility

Many DES children are now in their childbearing years and their experience is providing important data about the drug's effects on fertility. Researchers have discovered a spectrum of suspected and known DES side effects. Correlations to menstrual irregularities, decreased fertility, ectopic pregnancy, and early miscarriage are suspected. In some offspring known side effects include anatomical abnormalities of the reproductive organs that may cause pregnancy complications in DES daughters and decreased fertility in both DES-exposed men and women.

As a result of their prenatal exposure, some DES daughters have structural abnormalities of the vagina, cervix, or uterus. For example, the uterus may be "T" shaped or unusually small. Some DES daughters have problems with cervical mucus production, ovulation, conception or embryo implantation, miscarriage, premature deliveries, and tubal pregnancies. Many medical centers recognize these tendencies, carefully monitor DES-exposed pregnant women, and often refer them to premature labor prevention programs. It is important to remember, however, that an estimated 70 percent of DES daughters will have at least one successful pregnancy.

If you are a DES daughter or son concerned about health or fertility issues, it is important to find a specialist familiar with this drug and its long-term effects. A DES daughter should have a special examination periodically (as recommended by your physician) for careful scrutiny of the vagina and cervix, a complex Pap smear of all uterine quadrants, and perhaps a special test of the cervical cells.

CHAPTER 11

Endometriosis

► *Max had tears in his eyes. I asked him what the doctor had found. He only smiled and said he loved me very much. The doctor would be in soon to talk to me. Not such good news, I thought.*

It was one of the worst cases of endometriosis my surgeon had ever seen. My ovaries were grossly enlarged—nearly five times normal size. The Fallopian tubes were blocked and wrapped around my swollen ovaries. Endometriosis was in my large bowel as well. I had no chance of conceiving a child at present. With danazol therapy and surgery, I might have a chance.

I asked my doctor what could have happened if I had not sought help. He said that within the next year and a half, I would have been brought to emergency, bleeding internally and vaginally. I'd had endometriosis for probably 15 years, judging from its severity.

This disease is named after the endometrial cells, which normally compose the lining of the uterus and are expelled each month during menstruation. Endometriosis is caused by the growth of these cells outside the uterus—most typically in the ovaries and tubes (adnexa), the abdomen, or the exterior of the uterus—which would eventually damage the affected organs. In very rare cases, endometriosis has also been found in the lungs, heart, arms, and legs, and in the scars of previous cesarean sections.

As a disease entity endometriosis has been known to physicians for nearly 80 years. Knowledge about this condition has progressed with the development of gynecology as a subspecialty of general surgery. The more surgeons discover about endometriosis, however, the less they seem to understand it. Women who have the severest disease in terms of clinical findings (such as large cysts or massive scar tissue in the pelvis) may have very minor symptoms of pain and discomfort. Conversely, women with mild endometriosis can experience a lot of pain with menses and intercourse. The effect of endometriosis on fertility varies between patients.

Like uterine lining tissue, endometrial implants grow with the fluctuations of estrogen and progesterone hormones during the menstrual cycle. The body sometimes builds cysts (endometriomas or "chocolate cysts") around the foreign cells to confine them, temporarily preventing further invasion. About 60 percent of women with endometriosis develop endometriomas.

If not confined within cysts, endometriosis can grow freely on the reproductive organs and bleed painfully during menstruation. It is the inflammatory response of these implants that causes the pain associated with menstruation. This type of endometriosis may be more difficult to remove surgically.

The link between infertility and endometriosis has puzzled physicians. Only about 8 percent of women with endometriosis have blocked Fallopian tubes. Even when endometriosis is not directly affecting the tubes, ovaries, and uterus, however, there is often a problem in achieving pregnancy.

ENDOMETRIOSIS

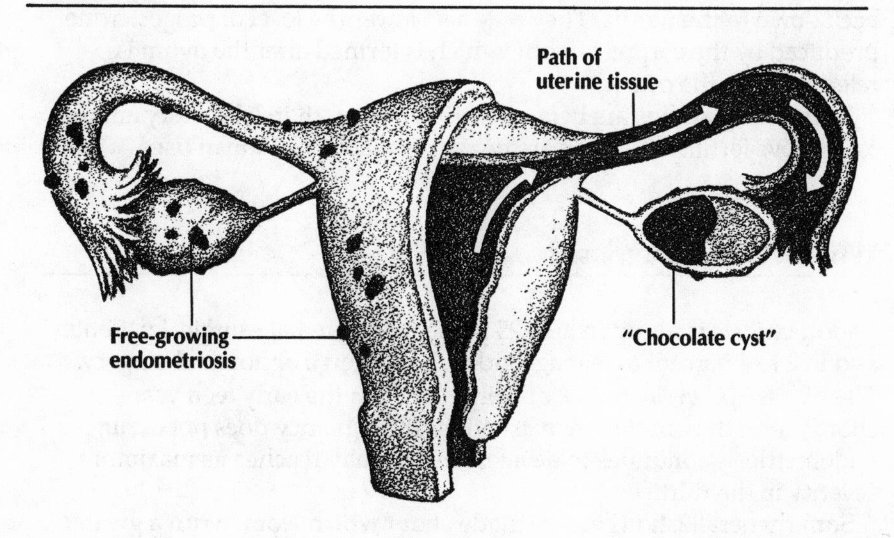

Emotional Effects

A diagnosis of endometriosis often foreshadows a chronic, painful, frustrating experience. Some women must face the consequences of this disease throughout their reproductive years: fertility problems, physical discomfort, frequent medical visits, and perhaps surgery or drug treatments. To cope with this problem, educate yourself about the disease and seek information from health professionals and reassurance and emotional support from other women who have endometriosis. For lists of further readings and support organizations, see the Selected Bibliography and Appendix A.

Causes

Although it is not known what causes endometriosis, one theory suggests that blood and endometrial cells occasionally back up through the uterus and tubes (retrograde bleeding) and attach to other reproductive organs.

Recent medical research has associated substances called prostaglandins with endometriosis. These pelvic fluids are released by the uterus before the menstrual period. One study found higher levels of prostaglandins in women with endometriosis than in other women.

Prostaglandins cause uterine contractions like menstrual cramps or labor pains. There is also speculation that they interfere with tubal motility, the rhythmic contractions of the tubes. This can impair the tube's ability to move the sperm up toward the ovum or the fertilized embryo back down to the uterus. They may also lower the level of progesterone produced by the corpus luteum, which is formed after the ovum is released from the ovary.

Antiprostaglandins are being experimented with in laboratory animals to improve fertility, but they are not yet available for human use.

Who Gets Endometriosis?

Endometriosis is found in 15 to 25 percent of all female surgical patients and in 2 to 4 percent of teenage girls who undergo abdominal surgery. The disease process probably begins slowly in the early teen years, shortly after the onset of menstruation. If pregnancy does not occur, endometriosis continues to develop and usually reaches its maximum severity in the thirties.

Some generalizations can be made about which women run a greater risk of developing this problem. Three-quarters of women suffering from endometriosis are between 30 and 40 years of age. Those who have experienced many years of menstrual cycles uninterrupted by pregnancy or lactation have a greater chance of developing this disease. Because more women are waiting to bear their children, the incidence of endometriosis is increasing. Endometriosis is found in about 20 percent of infertile women and seems to occur more often in those of higher socioeconomic background. It has also been suggested that endometriosis may be hereditary, but this theory has not been substantiated.

It is important to remember that these are only generalizations. *The medical profession does not know why some women develop endometriosis and not others.* Some literature has suggested that "overachieving," "aggressive," or "competitive" women are more likely to develop this problem. Such unscientific and unsubstantiated profiles are unfair and cruel explanations to offer to women confronting a painful and traumatic disease.

Symptoms

Symptoms of endometriosis include severe pain with menstruation or intercourse, particularly with deep penetration. When endometriosis occurs in other areas of the body, rectal pain with defecation, urinary tract burning, and abdominal pain may be experienced, depending on where the implants are located. Inability to get pregnant may occur in 40 percent or more of women with endometriosis. In fact the desire to become pregnant may bring a woman to the infertility workup that reveals the disease.

Diagnosis and Treatment

A pelvic examination and a medical history that includes irregular, painful, or heavy periods may suggest endometriosis. Occasionally nodules can be felt by physical examination at the back of the uterus. Although a hysterosalpingogram is an important diagnostic test to check the condition of the Fallopian tubes, it is usually not a reliable test for the presence of endometriosis.

Most physicians feel it is necessary to perform a laparoscopy to diagnose endometriosis. This procedure is often used to examine the intraabdominal area of patients who have pain or undetermined problems. It carries the risks of general anesthesia and surgery and there may be rare cases of bleeding, infection, or bowel perforation.

Although there is no known cure for endometriosis, it can be treated by surgically removing the implants or arresting their development with drug therapy. After treatment there is hope that the reproductive organs will again function normally and pregnancy will occur. Refer to Chapter 10 for a discussion of microsurgery. The following sections examine issues of surgical treatment appropriate to endometriosis.

Surgery by Laparoscopy

Microsurgery for mild endometriosis, sometimes called powder burns, can often be performed through the laparoscope. Adhesions can be cut, cauterized, or removed with a laser. Even quite extensive surgery can sometimes be performed during laparoscopy.

Major Surgery

Major surgery is often necessary to remove extensive endometriosis and any ovarian cysts or adhesions it has formed. Often such adhesions "glue down" the ovaries and tubes, preventing them from performing their natural functions.

Some surgeons prescribe danazol or oral contraceptive therapy before surgery to maximize their effect. During the operation a slippery liquid called dextran may be placed in the abdomen to prevent the organs from adhering to each other. Immediately after surgery, some physicians administer drugs intravenously while the patient is still hospitalized to prevent adhesion formation. Antibiotics are commonly used to fight infection.

Recurrence of Endometriosis or Adhesions After Surgery

If a pregnancy does not occur within a year or two, another laparoscopy is often recommended to reassess the situation. Unfortunately the first surgery itself may cause adhesions since the body often forms scar tissue while healing.

Surgery does not cure the disease. Endometriosis can and does recur in nearly 50 percent of patients within five years of treatment. It is recommended that pregnancy be attempted as soon as possible after surgery or drug treatment. Pregnancy rates are highest within the first two years after treatment and then decline.

Drug Therapy

► *For seven months I consumed four capsules of danazol daily. My horrendous periods stopped the first month of therapy. That was the good part. The worst part was that I gained 30 pounds and grew hair on my face.*

► *I have taken danazol for five months. I have not gained any weight or experienced any other negative effects. In part I attribute my feeling of good health to the absence of menstrual periods which, since the age of 11, have always been painful and nauseating. Secondly, the pressure to get pregnant is gone. Our sex life has improved because we again have sex when the mood strikes us, rather than when a schedule tells us.*

Danazol (brand name Danocrine) or oral contraceptives are sometimes used to treat endometriosis. Danazol, derived from a male hormone, acts directly on the ovaries, reducing their hormonal output to continuous, flat levels. Ordinarily the fluctuations of these hormonal levels create menstrual cycles. Ovulation and menstruation stop while danazol is taken. Although drug therapy does not remove existing scar tissue or ovarian cysts, it can arrest the disease temporarily so pregnancy can be attempted. Patients' reactions to danazol, as well as to oral contraceptives, vary tremendously.

Unfortunately side effects from danazol are fairly common. They include weight gain, possible abnormal hair growth on the face and chest, and deepening of the voice. Abnormal hair growth and voice changes may remain even after the drug is stopped. Some women also experience vaginal spotting and bleeding caused by changes in the uterine lining. If symptoms become severe, most physicians and their patients agree to stop danazol treatment. It is hoped that the lower dosages now being prescribed will reduce the occurrence of these problems.

Danazol is an expensive drug, costing over $100 per month on average. Most physicians prescribe danazol therapy for four to eight months. Then the patient is given an opportunity to get pregnant. The therapy may be prescribed again if pregnancy does not occur.

Oral contraceptives are also used to treat endometriosis. They stop ovulation, although menstruation occurs when the monthly cycle of pills is completed. Their cost is about one tenth that of danazol and their side effects are usually milder. Unlike danazol, however, the use of birth control pills carries a small risk of blood clotting problems. To date there have been no studies comparing the effectiveness of danazol and oral contraceptive therapy.

EFFECTIVENESS OF DRUG THERAPY FOR OVARIAN ENDOMETRIOSIS In ovarian endometriosis scar tissue often binds the ovary to the side wall of the pelvis or to the Fallopian tube and partially covers it. Even if the patient is ovulating, that envelope of scar tissue can block the ovum from entering the tube.

Endometrial implants, from 2 millimeters to 6 inches or larger in size, may also be present in large cysts within the ovary. Drug therapy is usually not effective in cysts more than 2 centimeters in diameter. The cyst will continue to grow and may leak endometriotic tissue elsewhere in the pelvis or cause discomfort and pain during the menstrual cycle. Surgery is usually more successful than drug therapy in treating ovarian endometriosis.

Pregnancy Rates Following Surgery and Drug Treatment

Pregnancy is an excellent treatment for endometriosis. Menstruation is halted for nine months or longer and often the endometrial implants shrink and disappear. Unfortunately endometriosis often impairs fertility and only half the women treated for this disease will experience a successful pregnancy.

One study, conducted over a ten-year period, compared patients who embarked on drug therapy with those who had surgery. Those who chose surgery had a slightly higher pregnancy rate.

CHAPTER 12

Immunological and Unexplained Infertility

► *After many tests our specialist found we had a sperm antibody problem. He wasn't sure if this was causing our long-term infertility or not, but it was the only problem ever diagnosed. He suggested we might use a condom for six months and then try to get pregnant again, or we could consider intra-uterine insemination. It's frustrating that so little is known about sperm antibodies, and it's difficult to find other infertile couples with this problem.*

► *We've tried to get pregnant for six years without success. Both of us have been tested and no physical problem was ever found. Some people who hear this are quick to say, "Well then, your infertility must be psychological."*

That's so unfair and so painful to hear. No one wants a baby more than we do.

Immunological Infertility (Sperm Antibodies)

The presence of sperm antibodies (immunological infertility), which can occur in both men and women, may contribute to or cause fertility impairment in 5 to 10 percent of infertile couples. Immunological infertility has, however, generated a great deal of controversy in the medical community. Experts disagree about the effects of sperm antibodies on fertility and about which couples should be tested or treated. Many researchers now think the presence of antibodies reduces the likelihood of pregnancy but does not prevent it.

Antibodies are protein substances (immunoglobulins) that are produced by the body's immune system and attack and destroy foreign cells. In most cases they protect us from illness. Unfortunately, antibodies sometimes consider sperm as foreign cells. In these cases they attach themselves to the sperm and cause problems with motility or penetration of an ovum.

Sperm antibodies can appear in the blood of both men and women and may also be present in the cervical mucus, uterine lining, Fallopian tubes, or semen. To confuse matters they may appear in the blood but not in the reproductive tract and vice versa; or there may be low levels of antibodies in the blood and high amounts in the cervical mucus or semen. Antibodies present in the reproductive tract are more likely to affect fertility.

Causes

It is thought that some women's immune systems develop antibodies after prolonged exposure to sperm. In some cases a temporary development of immunoglobulins may also result from an infection or intrauterine insemination (IUI). (IUI may trigger antibody formation by placing a greater amount of sperm in the tubes or uterus than normally occurs after intercourse.) In either case this allergic reaction probably exists toward all sperm rather than just those of one partner.

The occurrence of sperm antibodies in men is poorly understood. It is known that sperm occasionally wander out of the reproductive tract into the blood and cause an immune reaction. In fact 50 to 75 percent of men who have had a vasectomy will have measurable sperm antibodies afterward. Yet those antibodies frequently disappear after a vasectomy reversal or, if they remain, may not impair fertility.

Effect on Fertility

The degree of fertility impairment may depend on the type of antibody developed, its reaction to the sperm, and its concentration in the reproductive tract. In addition the place where the antibody attaches to the surface of the sperm seems to be critical. Although those attached to the end of the tail don't seem to hinder motility, antibodies that adhere to the main section of the tail can decrease or halt its movement through the cervical mucus. Those that attach to the head of the sperm can affect its ability to penetrate the outer covering of an ovum.

Testing for Immunological Infertility

When no other organic cause can be found for a couple's infertility during the workup, the specialist may recommend testing for sperm antibodies in both partners. It may also be appropriate to screen men considering a vasectomy reversal, couples whose postcoital or cervical mucus penetration tests show clumping or immobilization of sperm, and those considering in vitro fertilization (IVF).

In the past, several laboratory tests have been used to detect sperm antibodies in either partner. Semen was mixed with blood and/or cervical mucus in a test tube and the incidence of clumping (agglutinization) or immobilization was observed. A positive result was reported if 10 percent or more of the sperm reacted to the antibodies.

A more sophisticated test called the immunobead binding test has recently been developed. In this test the sperm are washed from the ejaculate and centrifuged. They are then mixed with microscopic beads that have been coated with antihuman antibodies (usually taken from a rabbit). The sperm are studied to note which antibodies have developed, where they have attached to the sperm's surface, and the percentage of total sperm with antibodies. This important information can give the specialist a better idea of how or why the antibodies are impairing the couple's fertility. If 50 percent or more of the sperm react to the antibodies, or if antibodies are attaching to the heads and upper tails of a significant number of sperm, a couple may be diagnosed with immunological infertility. A positive result, however, does not necessarily indicate this is the sole, or even a contributing, cause of the couple's infertility.

Treatment

The indications for and effectiveness of treatment for immunological infertility also generates controversy among medical experts. Some specialists think the treatments discussed below are worth a try in a case of sperm antibodies; others are skeptical of their effectiveness.

When the antibodies occur in the female partner, the couple may be advised that for a period of 6 to 12 months they should use a condom each time they have intercourse. This treatment presumes that the female partner's immune system will relax once the sperm are removed from her reproductive tract. When sperm are later reintroduced, it is hoped that antibodies will not form at least for a while and pregnancy can occur. There is little evidence, however, that this treatment is effective in reducing the presence of antibodies. Although success rates of 40 to 50 percent have been reported, these studies have been criticized for poor scientific methodology and controls.

Cortisone, which suppresses the immune system, may also be prescribed, although its use can produce adverse side effects. Success rates of 20 percent have been reported, although methodology and controls have also been questioned in these studies.

Treating an antibody problem in the male is also difficult. Sometimes intrauterine insemination is attempted after the ejaculate is centrifuged, the seminal fluid poured off, and donor seminal fluid or a chemical solution added. Reported pregnancy rates are about 25 percent with this method.

Unexplained Infertility

In about 10 percent of infertile couples, no organic cause can be found for their problem. This is called unexplained or "normal" infertility, which is a particularly inept adjective: There is certainly nothing "normal" about infertility or the stresses and heartache it brings.

Unlike those with a specific diagnosis, couples with unexplained infertility cannot focus their energy on a specific medical problem or treatment. They don't know what they are fighting or when to give up hope for a pregnancy. Their friends and relatives often suggest their problem is stress-related or even psychological in nature. Among infertile couples, they are most likely to hear the infamous advice, "Just relax" or "Take a vacation—you'll be pregnant next month."

In some happy instances, pregnancy *will* spontaneously occur. Other couples try for years without any success. Although there is no specific treatment for this problem, many in vitro fertilization and gamete intrafallopian tube transfer programs are now accepting some couples with unexplained infertility. Other couples with this problem also consider the options of adoption or child-free living.

CHAPTER 13

Pregnancy Loss:

Medical Facts and Emotional Aftermath

► *I got pregnant shortly after beginning infertility testing. Our thrill was short-lived as we lost the baby in the eighth week. This has been the most difficult part of our infertility.*

Some memories fade, but I can remember the days preceding my miscarriage very clearly. I still remember how stunned I was when I went to the bathroom and saw blood. That shocked feeling was so overpowering. I just sat there in that restroom for several minutes, then went to my sisters to seek reassurance that they had both spotted during their successful pregnancies.

The next three days were an agony. Finally one night I began bleeding heavily and passing clots. I made two trips to the emergency room with my husband only to be told to wait and expect cramps. I was not at all prepared for the intensity of the pain which was actually labor. It was 4 A.M. and I hadn't slept all night. I kept rationalizing what the pain could be. I knew an aspirin would help but thought it would be bad for the baby. I had to go to the bathroom but was afraid if I got up I would miscarry. That is what happened. I sat on the toilet and it was all over.

My husband and I have no regrets about picking up and looking at what should have been our baby. It seemed perfectly natural to us to say hello, and goodbye, and I love you.

Infertility is usually associated with an inability to conceive. Some infertile couples, however, may conceive easily only to lose one or more pregnancies before term. Their fertility problem involves an inability to carry their pregnancy to a live birth. Pregnancy loss may occur through miscarriage, ectopic pregnancy, or stillbirth.

Miscarriage

► *For those who have been sheltered from death and have not suffered the loss of anyone close, it can be the greatest loss of your life.*

For many years pregnancy loss was a taboo subject rarely discussed by couples between themselves or even with their doctors. Even today many people are uncomfortable with this subject. Most physicians, however, recommend an honest discussion of the possibility of miscarriage and its early symptoms with couples considering pregnancy.

Pregnancy loss is often regarded as a rare event that "couldn't ever happen to me." Actually, miscarriage (medically termed *spontaneous abortion*) is a common occurrence. *More than 50 percent of conceptions do not continue past the first few weeks.* This loss may be expelled in a heavier-than-usual period that is only a day or two late. In such cases the woman may not even realize she was pregnant.

About *15 to 20 percent of confirmed pregnancies end in miscarriage,* with three-quarters of these losses occurring during the first trimester. In addition, there is a 1 to 2 percent occurrence of ectopic (tubal) pregnancy, and about 1 in 80 pregnancies end in a stillbirth.

For some women miscarriage is a sudden, unexpected shock. Others experience symptoms of impending miscarriage for several days or weeks before it actually occurs. Their breasts may lose their fullness and tenderness, and light spotting or bleeding may begin. One woman described it as "just not feeling pregnant anymore."

During a *threatened miscarriage,* vaginal staining or bleeding occurs but the cervix remains closed. Sometimes this bleeding stops after a few days, allowing the pregnancy to continue successfully. However, if heavy bleeding and cramping occur and the cervix dilates, miscarriage is usually inevitable. A *complete abortion* expels all fetal tissue from the uterus, usually over a period of several days. If the symptoms continue but the fetal tissue is not expelled from the uterus, it is termed an *incomplete abortion.* A *missed abortion* describes a similar situation where fetal tissue remains or the fetus has died in utero, but symptoms have subsided. A dilation and curettage (D & C) is usually required to remove incomplete or missed abortions.

Causes

Miscarriage usually occurs when the body senses an abnormality in the fetus and rejects it to end the pregnancy. Such first trimester miscarriages are usually random events. An abnormal egg or sperm, a faulty union between them, or a chance mutation during early gestation is probably responsible, and the odds are heavily against a recurrence. Most specialists do not consider one or even two miscarriages an indication of any physical or hormonal problem.

However, there can be other causes of miscarriage. An insufficient uterine lining, caused by abnormal hormonal levels, may not properly nourish the embryo during early pregnancy, and an early miscarriage may result. Infection, some kinds of disease, smoking, and environmental toxins can also cause early miscarriage.

Second trimester miscarriages, on the other hand, are unusual. These are both emotionally traumatic and physically exhausting because the woman usually goes into labor. They can be caused by weakened cervical muscles or by anatomical abnormalities or tumors of the uterus. Immunological factors may also cause a woman's body to reject a second trimester pregnancy.

Repeated Miscarriages

Many women experience one or two miscarriages and then carry several successful pregnancies. There are, however, those who suffer three, four, or more pregnancy losses without carrying a child to term. Understandably, these women and their mates experience enormous grief and often view pregnancy as a frightening prospect.

The risk of recurrent miscarriages in a woman who has lost two prior pregnancies is about 25 to 30 percent. The medical community terms a woman who suffers three or more consecutive miscarriages an *habitual aborter,* although the recurrence rate for future miscarriages is still around 33 percent. This rate is higher than the 15 to 20 percent overall incidence of spontaneous miscarriage for all clinically recognized pregnancies.

Recurrent miscarriages are sometimes caused by an abnormality in the husband or wife, rather than a chance maldevelopment caused by a faulty union of sperm and egg. Causes of persistent or habitual miscarriages can include chromosomal defects in one of the parents, uterine abnormalities, and hormonal or infection problems.

Women who have suffered more than two miscarriages, or a second trimester pregnancy loss, should consult an obstetrician experienced in the management of difficult pregnancies and/or habitual miscarriages before attempting to conceive again. Each woman who suffers recurrent miscarriages must be individually evaluated and treated. She and her husband may need medical advice regarding activity restriction, specialized nutrition, frequency of office visits, and additional financial costs. Their specialist may order blood tests to check for anemia and thyroid function and perhaps cultures for chlamydia, mycoplasma, and other organisms. Studies such as chromosomal determinations, visualization or X-ray of the uterine cavity, Rh compatability, laparoscopy, and hormonal evaluation of the menstrual cycle may also be indicated.

Treatment for recurrent miscarriage problems may include surgery or drug therapy with hormones and antibiotics. With appropriate treatment, about 80 percent of women who suffer from recurrent miscarriages subsequently experience a successful pregnancy.

Emotional Aftermath of Pregnancy Loss

► *I miscarried this morning. There will be no baby. The world seems flat, colorless. I cry. Cry harder. It does no good. I sit on the sofa and stare out the window. A young mother pushes a stroller down the street.*

We have to tell our family. I make my husband do the phoning. I'm so embarrassed, ashamed. I've let everyone down, especially my husband. Perhaps he should have married a younger woman. I pack the maternity clothes to send back to my sister. She phoned this morning to tell me she's pregnant again.

Why did I miscarry? A genetic defect? Abnormal hormone level? I question and requestion the doctor. The medical reasons are unclear and somehow not really important in the bleak aftermath of miscarriage. Miscarriage, I hear again and again, is a common occurrence. But cold statistics in no way numb the pain. According to my doctor some women view a miscarriage as a pregnancy that never was; others see it as the death of a child.

I wish I was one of the lucky ones. Now everything is a constant reminder. The crib goes to the basement, eventually to Goodwill. Even diaper commercials bring a flood of tears. My sister tells me to control myself. "After all, you were only two months pregnant." She's right, of course. I must be overreacting. Still I can't stop crying.

The doctor wants me to come back and see her if I'm not pregnant again in several months. I don't keep the appointment. I can't face all those pregnant women in the waiting room. Most of all, I can't face the fear now synonymous with a second pregnancy.

I seem to be bombarded by babies. It seems as if someone phones each week with news of another pregnancy or birth. Every day brings a new baby-related crisis, and seeing friends with children becomes impossible. Everywhere there are babies and pregnant women with toddlers in tow. Even going to the supermarket becomes an ordeal of grief.

The months slip away, but I still cry daily. My husband is understanding and supportive, but I'm sure he's getting tired of tears. It's been a year since my miscarriage —a year heavy with unfulfilled dreams and rememberings.

Some people think of miscarriage as nature's way of ending an abnormal pregnancy and experience little grief afterward. Others view pregnancy loss as the death of their child and a major life crisis. They may carry this pain for some time, even though successful pregnancies follow.

One or both mates often form a deep attachment to the baby as soon as pregnancy is confirmed and are unable to accept the possibility of miscarriage. They are truly *expecting* a child from the first weeks of pregnancy and the baby becomes the central focus of their life. Even though the due date is months away, they may fantasize the sex or eye color of their baby, pick out names, and buy clothing and furniture for the nursery. When the pregnancy ends, their hopes and dreams are shattered. If this is their first miscarriage, they are often unprepared for the intensity of their reactions.

► *My doctor asked me how I could grieve over a "blob." I answered that I grieved for my baby which I had lost. For four months I did nothing much but cry. I really didn't know why I was so depressed.*

Some couples grieve for their baby just as they would mourn the death of a living loved one. The thought that they may have other children is little comfort now. This special, beloved baby is gone and cannot be replaced with someone else. *It is a real loss they have the right to mourn.*

Our society often denies or downplays the intensity of pregnancy loss. To many people, the fetus is a nonperson and its loss a nonevent. Those who mourn are bewildered by this attitude, finding it difficult to express their grief to others. Burying these feelings, they experience depression or lethargy and do not recognize these reactions as grief.

Grief may begin with numbness and shock, followed by anxiety, tears, or depression. People and things related to pregnancy and babies may be especially painful and ubiquitous. Many women feel empty and hopeless, fearing they will never be pregnant again. Depression may last for months or longer. Some women become preoccupied with their loss and endlessly review the pregnancy, the first signs of trouble, the physical experience of the miscarriage, and their emotional reactions.

Mourning is a gradual process. At first there may be weeks of uncontrollable weeping and sadness, but these lessen with time. Colleagues, friends, and relatives may be confused by the length or depth of your grief. Try being honest with them about your feelings and ask for their understanding and patience.

After a while there will be more easy days than difficult ones. Reminders may continue to recall the sadness of your loss, but the daily, incessant grief passes. Many find it helpful to talk with others who have experienced pregnancy loss. It is a common occurrence; you'll be surprised how many of your friends and relatives have also miscarried. Private counseling can also be valuable in cases of deep, long-term grief.

Others find closure in formal rituals such as funerals, memorial services, or writing an epitaph for their child.

CONFLICT BETWEEN PARTNERS Some couples find that the miscarriage has affected the partners differently, and communication problems quickly surface.

► *My husband didn't show any emotion while I cried constantly. I misinterpreted that and thought he didn't care, that he didn't really want the baby. I was very angry with him.*

A woman often grieves immediately after a miscarriage. Coping with physical as well as hormonal changes, she may take time off from normal activities to convalesce and absorb the loss. For a man, an early pregnancy may seem a bit unreal. His wife is not "showing," they probably have not even heard the baby's heart beat, and his body is not going through any physical or hormonal changes. Although he is saddened by the loss, the pregnancy is not as real to him. Concerned about his wife's physical and emotional health, he may also suppress his grief, thinking someone has to remain strong. In an attempt to help his wife, he may voice the same cliches as others. Many wives misinterpret this effort and his "strong silence" as apathy about their loss.

In addition to dealing with the miscarriage's effect on their lives, the man is probably also working full-time. He may have to tell family and coworkers about their loss and cope with the questions and sympathy of others. Coming home may also be upsetting if his wife is miserable. His life, too, becomes pressured and unhappy on all fronts. It is little wonder that as their wives become stronger and their grief subsides, many men take their turn at "falling apart." Their buried grief now surfaces in the form of tears, depression, or anger. It may take months, perhaps as long as a year, for both partners to complete their mourning.

One or both mates may also be afraid to attempt another pregnancy. Although most physicians feel it is safe to conceive again three cycles after a miscarriage, the husband may be afraid to subject his wife to another physical and emotional loss. She may fear that the next pregnancy won't take and they'll go through this despair again.

GUILT

► *I can't even guess at how many times I tortured myself with the reminder that I had gotten pregnant before and didn't really want to be, and that must have been why I lost the baby and why I was unable to conceive again. I was being punished for taking my fertility for granted, for not being grateful enough when I had the chance, for assuming that I had a right to choose and control when I would become a mother.*

► *I have counseled women who have guilt feelings about their miscarriage caused by comments from unthinking acquaintances, such as "You really were too active," "I told you not to lift those boxes," and so forth.*

It's hard to absorb the loss, hear those comments, and not feel some guilt.

"Why did it happen to me? What did I do wrong? Was it because we made love the night before?" These are all common questions after a miscarriage. Knowing why can become an obsession. Seeking to put blame somewhere may seem important, and some couples place it on themselves. Thoughtless questions and comments from others often intensify feelings of blame and guilt.

Try to remember that most miscarriages are inevitable and not anyone's fault. If feelings of guilt persist, it may be advisable to talk to your physician about testing for physical problems and get professional counseling about your feelings before attempting pregnancy again.

CHANGES IN BODY IMAGE

► *I remember hating my body after my miscarriage and not wanting to appear sexually attractive to anybody. One day on the street some man made a comment about my body and I became very angry.*

After a miscarriage a woman experiences a number of psychological and physical changes. Shifting hormonal levels, for example, can cause moodiness and irritability. She may also be disappointed or disgusted with her body, regarding it as inferior or inadequate for failing to hold the pregnancy. Some women have difficulty adjusting to a nonpregnant state and have an eerie feeling that they are still carrying a child.

The physical changes following a miscarriage last for only a few weeks. The body usually returns to its normal state, and menstrual cycles resume in about six weeks. Negative self-images, however, may last much longer.

REMARKS OF FAMILY AND FRIENDS

► *With all good intentions I was told by many that I shouldn't feel too bad about the miscarriage because I could always get pregnant again—as if Pinky had not been a real person to us; as if our dreams and hopes and plans had never existed.*

"There will be other children. It was meant to be. Something was wrong with the child. It's all for the best." These are sentiments usually offered after a miscarriage. Although well-intentioned, such remarks may not comfort the couple at all. Instead they convey the message that there is no cause for grief or depression. "It all happened for the best" is a particularly painful cliche. The couple wanted a baby and now they don't have one. The baby didn't get a chance to live. It is hard to see how that is for the best.

Instead of cliches, couples who have suffered a miscarriage need validation of their feelings and permission to express them. By recognizing its importance they can face their loss squarely and complete their grieving.

A frank discussion with close friends and relatives may benefit everyone. Let them know what helps and what hurts in terms of discussion, social events, visits, and so forth. You may also need to establish some physical and emotional distance from those who remain insensitive.

OTHERS' PREGNANCIES

► *I remember a close friend having a baby around the time of my miscarriage. I called her at the hospital and wished her well, but asked her not to call me or ask me to come see the baby.*

Envy and jealousy of pregnant friends and relatives is a common reaction after a miscarriage. They have something you wanted so badly but lost. At the same time you may feel happiness and excitement for them. Some women also have a superstitious fear of passing their misfortune on to their pregnant friends. These ambivalent emotions can be confusing and frightening.

Try to examine your feelings and reactions. Does the idea of socializing with pregnant friends seem overwhelming? You may want to call, express your feelings, and ask for their understanding while you grieve. Some couples decide not to socialize with these acquaintances for awhile, while others choose to limit their contact to those pregnant friends sensitive to their loss.

PREGNANCY LOSS AFTER INFERTILITY

► *I tried for nine years to get pregnant and just lost a baby two months ago. I am scared to join a miscarriage support group, because they're all fertile people who have lost babies but have this gleam of hope. I, on the other hand, am not sure if I do have another chance.*

Infertile couples, after spending years trying to conceive, are often devastated when a pregnancy loss occurs. They often feel this was their only chance at pregnancy and they "blew it."

It is also difficult for these couples to find emotional support. Many of their infertile friends have never experienced pregnancy or miscarriage, and most couples who miscarry will be able to conceive again. For empathy and reassurance, your physician or RESOLVE may be able to refer you to others who have suffered a pregnancy loss after long-term infertility.

TRYING AGAIN AFTER A PREGNANCY LOSS

► *My fears of having another miscarriage never really disappeared, even though my next pregnancy was anxious but uncomplicated.*

Those who try to conceive after a pregnancy loss are a little wiser and sadder. These women have lost not only their babies, but also the innocent elation others feel with the first news of pregnancy. They know about miscarriage firsthand and realize it can happen again.

To increase your chances for success, be sure to give your body enough time to recover from fatigue, blood loss, and any anemia that may have resulted from the miscarriage. Most physicians advise a three-cycle wait before conceiving again. With these precautions, you have a 70 percent chance for a successful pregnancy if no other fertility problem is present in either partner.

Most women feel anxious until they pass the point in pregnancy at which they lost their first baby—be it 6, 10, or 20 weeks or birth. Expect to feel concerned and uneasy until then. You will probably have more than the usual amount of fears with this pregnancy. This is also an anxious time for your mate; take care to comfort and support each other.

Try to enjoy your pregnancy as much as possible. Work closely with your obstetrician and call whenever you feel concerned. You may also want to talk with other couples who have experienced successful pregnancies after a miscarriage.

REPEATED PREGNANCY LOSSES

► *As I write this I am pregnant for a fifth time. My first four pregnancies ended in miscarriage. I have told only a few people. I know that I cannot bear to hear people say, "Oh, how wonderful! Congratulations!" It is impossible to convey to most of them that no, it is not wonderful, at least not at this point; that being pregnant is frightening and anxiety-producing and a situation in which daily life feels like walking on eggs.*

My husband and I rarely talk about this baby. We don't really allow ourselves to think of "it" as a baby yet. I am superstitious and in a state of emotional neutrality. I am merely waiting. It is not a pregnancy celebrated and enjoyed.

Yet way deep down, there is a very secret, very private place that all the self-protective, insulating behavior does not seem to penetrate. Tiny, light-filled fantasy images scamper out for whole moments at a time before they are ruthlessly squelched and shoved back inside the dark recesses of safety. "Will she have a funny, lopsided smile like her father's? Will I nurse him here by this window?"

Hope is always there, in little glimmers, impossible to deny. Yet, like a general marshaling huge armies, I fortify against those feelings. When, and only when, I hold that baby in my arms, will I allow myself to feel that pent-up explosion of joy.

Unlike those who cannot conceive, women who repeatedly miscarry may begin their pregnancies easily. Then time and again, perhaps only weeks after confirmation of their pregnancy, they miscarry. This is a heartbreaking problem that brings grief and fear with each loss.

If you habitually miscarry, seek a medically competent and emotionally supportive specialist who is experienced with high-risk pregnancy. Before you try to conceive again, the specialist may suggest preliminary tests or preventive treatment. Frequent office visits may be necessary to monitor the baby's development and your own health. To ensure a successful outcome some women may also require bed rest or hospitalization for part or all of their pregnancy.

It is important to have realistic expectations about your future pregnancies and seek emotional support from others with this problem. There is, however, new hope for women who repeatedly miscarry. Technological advances in the field of high-risk obstetrics are helping more of these women achieve successful pregnancies. Hopefully, with competent medical care and strong emotional support, you will also succeed.

Ectopic Pregnancy

► *First, there were the gas pains, sharper than any I'd ever experienced. Brief episodes at first, then a later, all-night episode that drove me crawling to my medical textbooks.*

"Ectopic pregnancy . . . the pain is frequently of colicky variety and in one of the lower abdominal quadrants . . . It frequently disappears for some hours or days before rupture occurs, only to reappear."

My physician's face was easy to read: "I think you have an ectopic. I'm afraid the only thing we can do is surgery. When did you last have something to eat?"

Surgery now . . . today . . . no time to prepare.

In many ways, the immediate postop period was easy. There was no more worry about an uncertain diagnosis. The pain was definite in origin, the surgery showed the remaining tube to be normal, allowing me denial of the full impact of the event. Of course there would be future pregnancies and children. But when alone in my room, I felt a bottomless emotional pain. The only baby that my husband and I ever made, that I had conceived, was gone. My right Fallopian tube, a part of my childbearing apparatus, was gone too. My body had been cut open to remove them. I felt empty.

My husband shared the loss in many ways. He spent the nights in the hospital with me, sleeping on a cot. Once we were home, he bandaged my incision daily, enabling me to shower. We exhaustively discussed and reviewed what had happened.

Talking with other women who had experienced ectopics was invaluable. I've been surprised at how much alike our reactions have been. All have described grieving periods of several months duration, feelings of lowered self-esteem and femininity, and serious concerns regarding our ability to have future children, despite medical assurance of our probable fertility.

Not so helpful were the frequent well-meaning comments from others such as, "Everything will be fine, you only need one tube"; "I think if I'd had an ectopic pregnancy, I'd be over it by now"; or "It may be a blessing in disguise; there could have been something wrong with the baby."

Ectopic pregnancy involves multifaceted loss: of the baby that would have been; perhaps of a valued body part (the Fallopian tube); and of self-esteem and femininity. Because it does not always result in sterility, the impact of reduced fertility is often not acknowledged by others. The decreased fertility was real to us, even if a successful pregnancy eventually occurs.

In about 1 percent of all pregnancies, a fertilized egg will implant somewhere outside the uterus. Usually this occurs in one of the Fallopian tubes. Such a pregnancy is termed ectopic or tubal. While it remains in the tube, an ectopic will result in a positive HCG serum pregnancy test and cause basal body temperature to remain elevated.

The fetus can grow only for a few weeks in this tiny area. As the tube stretches to accommodate the growing embryo, severe abdominal pain is experienced. If the pregnancy is not removed, the tube will rupture. The resulting internal bleeding and attendant shock create a life-threatening condition.

Ectopic pregnancy requires immediate, competent medical care. It is critical to seek help before a rupture occurs. If the ectopic is caught early, the surgeon may be able to remove the fetus and save part or all of the affected Fallopian tube.

Although any woman can develop an ectopic pregnancy, there does seem to be a higher incidence among those who have used IUDs or have tubal adhesions or scarring resulting from pelvic inflammatory disease or previous tubal surgery. Only 50 percent of women who have had an ectopic pregnancy will conceive again, and 10 percent of them will suffer another tubal pregnancy.

Ectopic pregnancy evokes many of the same reactions as miscarriage. It also is a critical condition that requires emergency surgery and many women lose part or all of a Fallopian tube during the procedure. It is common to feel depressed, angry, and empty after losing part of your body. After an ectopic many couples are afraid to attempt pregnancy again. This has been both a miscarriage and a life-threatening emergency.

Stillbirth

SONG OF SAMANTHA

God, my baby is gone, gone—
where I cannot go,
Gone where I cannot care for her
as I did
She grew inside me, now they tell me
she's stillborn
Still, still, still..they tell
me she's dead,
Not waiting down the hall, not
needing me any more.
Still, still, still she is
my baby
And my tears fall like rain.
My belly is empty but I am alone.
She came but did not stay
and my tears fall like rain.
Others have theirs, but my baby
is gone
And my tears fall like the rain.

(Brochure on stillbirth, by Ronna Case, Chaplain, Eskaton American River Hospital)

Stillbirth is a heartbreaking conclusion to pregnancy. Occurring about once in every 80 births, it is defined as the death of a fetus in the third trimester of pregnancy or during labor and delivery. Some women discover their baby has died in utero during their last trimester, perhaps during a routine prenatal visit. They may have an agonizing wait of several days or longer before labor begins or is induced. Other women begin normal labor fully prepared to deliver a healthy, live baby. They may learn of the baby's death during labor or upon delivery.

In cases of in utero death detected before delivery, some women and their physicians decide to use general anesthesia for the birth; others opt for a milder anesthetic or even natural childbirth. Afterward the woman's body goes through postpartum changes: Her hormones readjust and her breasts fill with milk as she tries to absorb the loss of her child.

The first and most agonizing question after stillbirth is "Why? What made this happen?" In some cases anoxia (lack of oxygen), umbilical cord dysfunction, toxemia, or diabetes may affect the growth and health of the fetus. The placenta may separate from the uterus (*abruptio placentae*), or implant between the baby and the cervix (*placenta previa*). Infection caused by the waters breaking too early or too stressful a labor can also be contributing factors. Unfortunately, however, the cause of death cannot be determined in nearly half of the stillbirths that occur.

Grieving and Coping

► *Often I struggle with my memories of the stillbirth. I couldn't keep all the emotions filed and bottled inside. I am thankful we had close friends outside our immediate family to talk to. But mostly it helped to talk with my wife. I found that sharing our feelings with each other brought us closer together than we had ever been. We had planned together for our child, prepared ourselves for the new addition, dealt with the pregnancy for nine months, decorated the nursery together. Yet our baby was gone.*

Stillbirth carries all of the aftermath of other pregnancy losses plus its own unique pain. The couple must deal with many intense emotions in quick succession, including the shocking discovery that the baby has died in utero or during delivery. This death is totally unexpected and they usually do not have time to absorb and accept the loss before it occurs.

Following the stillbirth, both parents experience deep grief at a time when difficult decisions must be made. A death certificate must be completed to be signed by the physician. In most cases the couple must decide whether to view or hold their child, give their baby a name, and take his or her picture. Someone must notify relatives and friends and make funeral or burial arrangements.

The following suggestions may help the couple deal with the immediate aftermath of their stillbirth and the grieving period that follows:

- Ask for a private room on another floor of the hospital. If your request is refused, remain adamant and enlist your doctor's help if necessary. Changing floors will remove you from newborns and their delighted parents.

- Ask your physician and one of the floor nurses to inform other medical personnel, on the maternity wing and at your new location, about your loss. This may spare you from explanations to nurses, lab technicians, and physicians unaware of your tragedy.
- Some couples prefer to spend as much time together as possible to comfort and support each other. Most hospitals will put a cot in the room so your husband can remain with you overnight. Other women and men, when in the midst of deep grief, need solitude. If your mate is overwhelmed by the death and temporarily unable to offer consolation, call on trusted family or friends to stay with you.
- To soften another surge of grief, you may request a shot to dry up the milk that comes in a few days after the birth. If you prefer not to use medication, bind your breasts and apply warm compresses to ease the pain until the milk dries up. This usually takes several days.
- Discuss whether you want to see or hold the baby. One partner may wish to and the other may not. Some couples prefer that their mother, father, or another loved one view their child for them. Most hospitals take a picture of the baby and keep it in a file. It is comforting to know you can request it at any time.
- You don't have to bear your grief alone either now or in the months to come. Seek emotional support and assistance from trusted friends and relatives. There are also organizations staffed by those who have experienced stillbirth (see Appendix A). You can call them at any time of the day or night for solace and support.

CHAPTER 14

The New Frontiers:

In Vitro Fertilization, Gamete Intrafallopian Tube Transfer, and Embryo Transfers

► *"You must be kidding!" That was my comment when our infertility specialist told my husband and me that IVF was a real option for having a second biological child. The physician's recommendation was the culmination of three years of fighting the infertility battle. Those years included the diagnosis of blocked Fallopian tubes leading to tubal surgery, followed by an ectopic pregnancy and more tubal surgery. I was left with only two-thirds of one Fallopian tube and no baby.*

In 1978 the dramatic conception and birth of England's "test-tube" baby, Louise Brown, ushered in a new age of infertility technology. Since that miracle, in vitro fertilization (IVF) has been enthusiastically discussed and widely publicized. To date more than 4000 children worldwide have been born through IVF, more than 600 of them in the United States. Over the past several years, there has been a proliferation

of knowledge and a refinement of technique in IVF, and more pregnancies are occurring each month. Many programs have since opened both in the United States and abroad.

In addition, several other high-tech medical procedures have been developed to treat human infertility. Gamete intrafallopian tube transfer (GIFT) is a process in which one or more eggs are surgically removed from the ovary and then together with the mate's sperm, injected into the Fallopian tube for natural (in vivo) fertilization and implantation. In the embryo transfer process, an egg that was fertilized through insemination with the husband's sperm is aspirated from a donor woman's womb and implanted into the uterus of an infertile woman.

These treatments are exciting scientific advances and offer some hope to infertile couples. They are, however, still in their earliest stages of development, and their success rates are discouragingly low. For most couples, these techniques will ultimately be another stressful and expensive disappointment. It is hoped that with further research and experience these high-tech advances will hold a brighter promise for future infertility treatment.

These new frontiers of treatment also pose controversial ethical and moral questions. The very term *test-tube* baby recalls Aldous Huxley's vision of the frightening, futuristic society of *Brave New World*. Everyone seems to be talking about IVF and other advances these days, and the ethics of these procedures are hotly debated by politicians, theologians, scientists, feminists, physicians, and infertility patients.

Should fertilization of human eggs be performed in a laboratory? How much should we control and interfere with biological processes? Are men and women being treated in a caring, humane manner? Is IVF an ethical and appropriate treatment? Should it be available only to the affluent or those with enough insurance coverage? What are the lifelong effects of this procedure on babies conceived this way? Should fertilized embryos be "frozen" for indefinite periods of time? Should "unused" embryos be discarded or donated to other infertile couples?

In the late 1970s the Department of Health, Education, and Welfare investigated the ethics of offering IVF in the United States. Although its report endorsed the practice of IVF under certain conditions, it did not recommend federal funding for treatment and research. The American Fertility Society has also endorsed the practice of IVF in the United States under specified conditions.

Despite this controversy, numerous IVF clinics have opened in the United States, and more successes are being reported. GIFT and embryo transfer programs are also becoming available to infertility patients. Still the debate rages, and the pioneers of these new technologies—the patients and their medical teams—receive both praise and criticism from an ambivalent society.

In Vitro Fertilization

In vitro fertilization is a highly technical, complex process that involves ovulation induction through fertility drugs, removal by surgery or ultrasound technique of one or more eggs from the mother, and fertilization of those eggs with the father's sperm in a plastic dish. (*In vitro* literally means "in glass," but plastic dishes are now commonly used.) The fertilized embryo is then incubated and transferred into the mother's uterus with the hope of a successful pregnancy and birth.

This monumental medical breakthrough was neither easily achieved nor a result of luck. Dr. Robert Edwards, a British reproductive physiologist, has researched IVF with human eggs since 1963. He began collaborating with Dr. Patrick Steptoe, a British obstetrician, more than a decade before the first birth occurred.

Unquestionably IVF is an exciting medical treatment, renewing hope for many infertile couples who do not respond to surgical or drug treatment. But IVF is surrounded by a great deal of myth and misunderstanding. The unsolicited advice offered to infertile couples now has a new twist: "Don't worry. You can always have a test-tube baby!"

In fact this is usually the last resort for many couples who have already endured years of unsuccessful medical treatments and surgeries that offered higher success rates than IVF. Their remaining shreds of hope now focus on this final medical effort. It is an extremely stressful experience, and *only 10 to 20 percent of IVF attempts culminate in a live term pregnancy.*

Infertility specialists strongly urge any couple or single woman considering IVF to research the procedure carefully before making a decision. In this way they enter the IVF process aware of its physical, financial, psychological, and emotional demands and have a realistic idea of their chances for success.

Indications for IVF

IVF may be recommended to a couple for a variety of infertility problems:

- Tubal blockages or adhesions. In many cases the first try with microsurgery still yields higher success rates than IVF. If, however, a pregnancy does not occur within two years of the microsurgery, IVF may be an appropriate option. In cases of tubal abnormalities, some specialists feel that IVF is less physically traumatic and less expensive and offers better success rates than repeated microsurgery.

- Endometriosis that does not respond to surgical or medical treatment. Again, IVF may be more successful and less invasive than repeated surgical attempts.
- Infertility traced to sperm antibodies.
- Some types of male infertility, such as low sperm count, and cases where fertility drug treatment has not resulted in pregnancy.
- Long-standing unexplained infertility, in which no physical problem can be found in either partner.

Making the Decision

The success rates, as well as the physical, emotional and financial demands of IVF, must be carefully weighed before a couple or single woman decides on this option. Most couples have already been through several years of infertility stress and treatment; many women have undergone major surgery. This experience will again stress an already taxed relationship.

Age must also be considered. Fertility naturally declines as women reach their thirties and forties and affects IVF success rates. Women over 35 should also consider the higher incidence of birth defects such as Down's syndrome for this age group and decide whether they are comfortable with such prenatal testing as amniocentesis.

Some questions you might consider before deciding on IVF include:

- Have you both read about the procedures, success rates, and requirements of the IVF process?
- Are you both willing to undertake the physical and emotional stress of this experience?
- Can you afford the expense of several attempts?
- Can you both handle the disappointment of an unsuccessful attempt?
- Are you agreed on how many times to try IVF before pursuing other options?
- Do you feel confident about the program selected?
- Are you getting enough emotional support? Should you seek private counseling while in the process?

IVF is a difficult physical and emotional experience and this option is not appropriate for everyone. *No one should feel pressured to try IVF.* There are other alternatives for every infertile couple, such as adoption or child-free living.

Selecting an IVF Program

► *We were living outside Washington, D.C. at the time, so my husband and I submitted an application and medical records to the Vital Initiation of Pregnancy (VIP) Program of the Eastern Virginia Medical School in Norfolk, Virginia. We were accepted for a diagnostic interview two months later. The odds were against us: There had been only two IVF babies born in the United States at that time, and there were only two or three IVF programs in the country that were fully operational. Yet it was difficult not to feel hopeful, not to believe that somehow our "lucky number" would come up.*

In the past several years, many IVF clinics have opened in the United States and around the world. Your specialist can advise you about various IVF clinics and their quality. RESOLVE also offers a current list of programs across the country. Call or write for detailed information about each program's guidelines, costs, and success rate.

Cost is an important consideration when selecting a program. Because the U.S. government does not provide funding for IVF or GIFT programs, each clinic must be self-supporting. Depending on the program, the 1987 cost for the IVF process ran between $3500 and $8000 per attempt. Most programs offer patients three or four tries at IVF.

Medical insurance coverage for IVF varies tremendously. Some carriers will cover all of the cost. Others will pay for only part of the expense. For instance the laparoscopy procedure is often considered "infertility diagnosis," and a percentage of that portion may be covered. Increasingly, however, insurance companies are refusing to pay for any part of an IVF procedure. (See Chapter 3 for a discussion of the economics of infertility.)

Many programs require that the entire cost be paid before each attempt. You may also have to travel some distance to an IVF program. Cost of travel, up to two weeks of accommodations, and perhaps wages lost from work should be added to the expenses.

You'll want to compare candidacy requirements, cost, waiting time, and success rates among programs. For further guidance, check the American Fertility Society's standards for IVF programs.

Requirements for IVF Candidates

Each IVF program has its own screening procedures and criteria for acceptance. All will require your previous medical records, infertility workup test results, and surgery reports. Most programs assume that the patient has exhausted other methods of medical treatment before attempting IVF. Some will require a preliminary laparoscopy to determine whether your ovaries are accessible for egg retrieval.

Most programs also require that applicants meet most or all of the following requirements:

- Ability to ovulate. The woman must be capable of ovulation, have at least part of one functioning ovary, and respond to the fertility drugs that will stimulate the formation of one or more eggs.
- Accessibility of ovaries. Some programs require that the patient have surgically accessible ovaries. This means that the surgeon can reach the surface of the ovary through laparoscopy, and puncture it with a needle to aspirate one or more mature follicles. Women who have extensive adhesions around the ovaries caused by endometriosis may not be immediate candidates for IVF. These women may require preliminary surgery to remove the adhesions and make the ovary accessible. (Tubal scarring, often caused by IUDs or pelvic inflammatory disease, should present no problem for IVF.)

  Other programs employ techniques that aspirate the egg through the bladder or vaginally through ultrasound. If you have ovarian adhesions, check with each IVF program about their aspiration techniques.
- Age. Most IVF programs will accept women up to age 40, and exceptions may be made for those between 40 and 44. Because there is some decline in fertility in the midthirties and early forties, some programs give priority to women over 35.
- Rubella immunity. Before IVF is attempted, it is wise to test for rubella immunity and be vaccinated if necessary. If the mother is not immune and contracts rubella during early pregnancy, birth defects could result.
- Male partner fertility. Presumably a complete semen analysis of the male partner was performed during the workup. In addition, the hamster egg test is usually done before an IVF attempt to check the sperm's ability to penetrate an ovum. (See Chapter 15 for further discussion of these tests.) IVF is also sometimes appropriate for male factor infertility. If this is not feasible, some programs will perform IVF using donor sperm.
- Counseling. Most programs require preprogram interviews, psychological evaluations, and/or counseling to assess the couple's ability to cope with the emotional and physical stress of the IVF experience. The process is usually described in detail, and the couple is informed of potential health risks and chances of success. In addition, they are urged to plan for alternative resolutions if IVF should not be successful. Few programs, however, have ongoing counseling and psychological

services available during the process. If you undertake IVF, you may want to arrange for emotional and psychological support.

The Medical Process of In Vitro Fertilization

The IVF process currently involves ovulation induction with fertility drugs, monitoring of follicular development, surgical removal and laboratory evaluation of ovum, semen collection, fertilization of the egg with sperm in a plastic dish, incubation of the developing zygote, transfer of the embryo back to the uterus, and perhaps hormonal support during the first few weeks of pregnancy or until menstruation occurs. This process takes about two weeks from initial induction of ovulation through fertility drugs to transfer of the fertilized embryo. Many IVF patients describe the process as a roller coaster of hope, impatience, exhilaration, disappointment, and sometimes despair.

TABLE 14.1 The In Vitro Fertilization Medical Process

The IVF process is both stressful and costly (1987 fees range from $4000–8000 per attempt, depending on the program and procedures used). At each step, many patients either drop out voluntarily or fail to respond to treatment and are unable to continue. Only 10–20 percent of those who begin are blessed with a live infant nine months later. The complete procedure follows these steps:

	Induce ovulation with Clomiphene and/or Human Menopausal Gonadotropin (HMG).
If patient ovulates,	monitor follicular development through blood tests and ultrasound.
If eggs develop,	retrieve ova by laparoscopy or through bladder or vagina.
If retrieval successful,	evaluate ova in laboratory for maturity.
If ova are fertilizable,	collect semen from male partner.
If semen collected,	culture and incubate ova and sperm.
If fertilization and normal cell division occur,	transfer fertilized eggs into patient's uterus.
	Perform pregnancy test after 10–14 day wait.
If **negative** (80–90 percent),	couple must decide whether to try again.
If **positive** (10–20 percent),	natural progesterone may be given during early pregnancy.
If miscarriage does not occur,	live term infant is born nine months later.

OVULATION INDUCTION WITH FERTILITY DRUGS

► *Our journey was by no means at an end when we visited the Norfolk program for the first time. At that time I was given a laparoscopy to check the "accessibility" of the ovaries, and an unsuccessful effort was made then to retrieve an egg on a natural cycle.*

The second time, I was started on a protocol, which included daily injections of HMG.

Most IVF programs use either clomiphene, HMG, or a combination of the two to stimulate the development of more than one egg (superovulation). An injection of HCG hormone to aid final development of the ovum is also usually required.

Using fertility drugs has two advantages. First they enable a more precise timing of ovulation. It is important to retrieve the egg from the ovary just before ovulation occurs: It cannot be fertilized if it is immature, and it is difficult to locate once it has been released from the ovary. Secondly superovulation usually stimulates the development of several eggs, which can be taken from the ovaries, fertilized outside the body, and transferred. This increases the chances that one of those eggs will successfully implant and develop.

Unfortunately, large doses of fertility drugs are often used during IVF treatment. These drugs may produce unpleasant physical and emotional side effects, an important factor to weigh when considering IVF treatment.

MONITORING FOLLICULAR DEVELOPMENT

► *Blood was drawn daily, and sonograms were taken to check follicle development on the ovaries and to determine the time of ovulation. Approximately 36 hours prior to ovulation I was given an injection of HCG, which would ultimately trigger the release of the eggs from the follicles. By that time I felt like a human pin cushion: My bottom became sore and I began taking hot baths each night to relieve the pain and, more importantly, to relax.*

Several methods are used to monitor the development of follicles, the fluid-filled sacs within the ovary that contain the eggs. After clomiphene or HMG is administered, daily blood tests are required to assess estrogen and LH levels. Cervical mucus, retrieved by pelvic examination, may also be tested to determine whether ovulation is imminent.

Ultrasound, the bouncing of high frequency sound waves from the ovary, is also done daily to track the growth of the follicle(s). In this painless procedure the woman lies comfortably on a table, her abdomen is coated with a lubricant, and an ultrasound instrument is passed over her pelvic area. Her reproductive organs become visible on a screen and a picture can be made of the developing follicles. Before the test the patient must drink four or more glasses of water to distend the bladder, which makes the ovaries more visible. The only discomfort is usually caused by a full bladder.

In a new method of ultrasound, vaginal scanning, a slender instrument is inserted into the vagina. This procedure, which takes only about five minutes to perform, does not even require a full bladder.

As the follicles mature, they secrete increasing amounts of estrogen. When blood tests show peak estrogen levels, an HCG shot is often given to further stimulate follicular development. Ovum retrieval by laparoscopy or ultrasound aspiration is usually scheduled within 36 hours of this injection. Daily visits to the clinic or hospital are required during this initial six to ten day period.

RETRIEVING THE EGGS

► *On that July visit five immature ova were retrieved through a laparoscopy. However, 72 hours after the egg retrieval, only one fertilized egg had divided satisfactorily and remained viable. Ten days after this egg was transferred back into the uterus I was given a pregnancy test. The results were negative.*

Most patients undergo a laparoscopy, a surgical procedure usually performed on an outpatient basis. After general anesthesia is administered, carbon dioxide gas is introduced into the abdomen to distend it. A puncture is made near the navel and the laparoscope is inserted. This instrument, which resembles a telescope with a light source at one end, enables the surgical team to visualize the ovary. A second instrument is used to stabilize the ovary, and then a fine needle is inserted into the follicle that contains the egg. The follicle is punctured, and the mature egg and about a teaspoonful of the surrounding fluid are withdrawn by suction.

If the patient's ovaries are not directly accessible because of severe endometriosis or ovarian adhesions, the IVF team may try to aspirate the follicles through the bladder (transvesically) or the vagina (transvaginally). These techniques eliminate the need for major surgery to remove the adhesions, but are less successful than aspiration by laparoscopy.

Most patients develop between one and three eggs; some produce many more. In about 90 percent of cases, the attempt to withdraw between four and five eggs is successful. The surgical team is rarely unable to retrieve at least one egg. Because there doesn't seem to be any advantage in transferring more than four embryos with each IVF try, the others may be frozen in liquid nitrogen and saved for a future attempt. This is a controversial procedure, and each program has its own policy about freezing ova or sperm.

EVALUATION OF OVUM The retrieved eggs are immediately evaluated, and the most mature follicles are selected for the fertilization attempt. Immature eggs may be incubated for 24 hours in the laboratory; the IVF process is then continued. There is no evidence that an immature ovum will adversely affect the pregnancy or baby.

SEMEN COLLECTION Most programs prefer a fresh semen specimen collected within five hours of the laparoscopy. The male partner is asked to abstain from ejaculation for a least 48 hours prior to the collection. He usually provides the semen through masturbation and is called to the clinic at the time of the laparoscopy. For many men, this is an anxiety-producing situation. Some programs will store a previously collected, frozen sample although success rates using fresh sperm are higher.

The couple usually leaves the hospital at this point to wait for the fertilization and incubation process to be completed and for the call to return for embryo transfer.

FERTILIZATION After the eggs are aspirated from the ovary, each is separately cultured in a plastic dish. A carefully balanced culture fluid, free of bacteria and with a specific chemical content, is used.

About six or seven hours later the sperm are added to each culture. An average ejaculate contains 300 million sperm. In the body (in vivo), only about 400 sperm reach the vicinity of the egg and usually only one will penetrate it. During IVF, between 50,000 and 500,000 sperm are added to each egg culture.

These cultures are then incubated under precise conditions of humidity at body temperature. The gas content of the air is also strictly controlled. For the next few days the cultures are closely observed to determine whether fertilization and cell division has occurred.

EMBRYO TRANSFER The fertilized eggs are now called zygotes. During normal reproduction a zygote immediately divides and continues to do so for four to five days as it travels down the Fallopian tube. When it reaches the uterus, it contains either 64 or 128 cells and is called a blastocyst.

During the IVF process, the zygote is allowed to divide for about two days, to the two- to eight-cell stage. Although an IVF zygote is significantly less developed when it reaches the uterus than its in vivo counterpart, pregnancy rates are highest when transfer is made two to three days after laparoscopy.

The embryo transfer is done at the clinic, usually on an outpatient basis. No anesthesia is required. The patient is prepped for a pelvic exam, a speculum inserted in her vagina, and her cervix cleaned. The fertilized embryos are immersed in a protein-enriched drop of culture fluid and placed in a catheter attached to a syringe. The catheter is threaded through the cervix and into the uterus, where the embryos are injected. After embryo transfer, most women remain in bed for 1 to 12 hours. Some programs advise their patients to draw their knees into their chests for a short time after the transfer. Occasionally a woman will be hospitalized overnight. Most women can resume normal physical activity about 24 hours later.

After embryo transfer, the couple must wait an endless 10 to 14 days before a pregnancy test can be done.

HORMONAL SUPPORT AFTER EMBRYO TRANSFER During normal fertilization the corpus luteum (the follicle remaining in the ovary after ovulation) secretes increasing amounts of progesterone hormone to sustain the pregnancy until the placenta can take over. Some IVF teams fear that the aspiration process affects the corpus luteum and its subsequent progesterone production. They believe the chances for successful pregnancy can be increased by hormonal support after the embryos are transferred. They administer natural progesterone, through suppositories or injections, for the first few weeks of pregnancy or until menstruation occurs.

SEX RATIO OF IVF BABIES Most of the earlier IVF babies were females. It is thought this occurred because clomiphene was used to induce ovulation. Now that HMG is also being used, the boy/girl ratio seems to be equalizing.

CESAREAN BIRTHS Many of the earlier IVF babies were delivered by cesarean section. This may have been because everyone involved was quite cautious about these pregnancies. The cesarean rate is declining as the IVF procedure is refined.

Success Rates

► *There were so many disappointments along the way. Was it worth all of the emotional and physical stress and anguish to try again? It took six months before I was able to answer that question in the affirmative. In February I found myself back in Norfolk. The protocol was essentially the same. Yet my attitude had changed. The previous two experiences had humbled me somehow. I knew my body better, it was something I could never take for granted. This time, four ova were retrieved, four fertilized and divided satisfactorily, and four were transferred! I was euphoric. Many of my fellow patients, as well as my friends at home, were ready to knit booties for us. Ten days following the transfer, I had a pregnancy test. The doctor called me with the results. To my disbelief and dismay, I was not pregnant.*

There is a great deal of confusion about interpreting the success rates of IVF programs. Some clinics report pregnancy rates as high as 30 percent. Others claim a 10 to 15 percent success rate.

Why is there such a discrepancy? Patients drop out of the program at each stage, some women do not respond to the fertility drugs and ovulation does not occur, and sometimes an egg cannot be aspirated during the laparoscopy. Statistics can also be skewed by including only women who successfully complete the transfer stage of IVF.

When pregnancy does occur, percentages can also be misleading. Some programs may report all pregnancies achieved in a sample of patients as successes and not adjust the figures for transient BBT rises or subsequent miscarriages and ectopic pregnancies.

When considering an IVF program, *determine how many live term births have resulted in relation to the number of patients entering the process.* For example, 1000 patients divided into 110 live term births equals an 11 percent success rate.

Among IVF programs, today's actual success rates range from about 10 to 20 percent. These are IVF pregnancies that result in a live term birth. The number of embryos transferred also affects the success rate. When only one embryo successfully divides and is transferred, rates are close to 10 percent. Implanting two embryos increases the chances to about 20 percent, and three or more implanted embryos may result in greater than 20 percent success rates. The chances for success are the same with each attempt.

OBSTACLES TO HIGHER SUCCESS RATES Most IVF programs boast an 80 to 90 percent success rate for ovum retrieval, fertilization, and cell division. The major obstacles to higher IVF success rates have been proper hormonal stimulation, successful implantation during the transfer stage, and early pregnancy loss.

Batches of HMG hormone vary and each woman responds differently to fertility drug stimulation. Thus many patients are unable to produce viable follicles to aspirate.

Implantation problems and early pregnancy loss may be partially caused by transferring an embryo that is less developed than one normally would be in vivo. Unfortunately implanting a two- to eight-cell embryo seems to yield a higher success rate than waiting until it has divided to the body's normal 64- to 128-cell stage.

Early pregnancy losses are also difficult to prevent. In fact many pregnancy losses occur naturally. If 100 ovulated eggs were exposed to sperm in vivo in women 25 years of age, only about 31 percent would produce a live birth. This success rate declines as a woman ages. In her midthirties, she has only a 15 to 20 percent chance of a successful term pregnancy resulting from unprotected intercourse. These odds decline further as she passes 40.

IVF is now approaching about half the body's success rate. It is doubtful that science will ever surpass Mother Nature, but hopefully a success rate comparable to the body's will be approached as the IVF technique is refined.

HOW MANY TRIES? There is usually no restriction on the number of times a couple can try IVF. Because of the financial and emotional stresses, however, most couples try only once or twice. Few couples attempt IVF more than three times. Most programs recommend at least one "rest cycle" between tries.

Risks of IVF

SURGERY Laparoscopy, performed under general anesthesia, is often used to retrieve the mature follicles from the ovary. Any surgical procedure and anesthesia carry some risks.

FETAL ABNORMALITIES The IVF pregnancy does run a higher-than-normal risk of an egg being fertilized by two sperm. Normally, when the egg and sperm unite, one set of 23 chromosomes is contributed by each parent (the diploid number). If two sperm fertilize the egg, three sets of chromosomes are contributed and an abnormal fetus results. There is a very strong mechanism in the body, however, that rejects such abnormal embryos.

There are six species of mammals in which IVF and embryo transfer have resulted in live births. In all six species, the number of normal IVF offspring has been encouraging and there is probably no significant risk of inducing fetal abnormalities with this process. Because children conceived through IVF are still fairly young, however, the long-term health risks of this procedure are still not known.

DES-RELATED RISKS With both in vivo and IVF pregnancies, DES daughters with uterine abnormalities run a greater risk of miscarriage or premature delivery. Some DES daughters also have an abnormally small cervical opening, which may make insertion of the catheter for embryo transfer more difficult.

ECTOPIC PREGNANCY With IVF there is a slightly higher chance (3 percent as compared to 1 percent in the general population) of an ectopic pregnancy. Even though the Fallopian tubes are bypassed during the IVF process, an ectopic pregnancy can occur when the tubal-uterine junction is damaged and the embryos float back into the Fallopian tube and implant. Another theory, difficult to prove, suggests that excess force or fluid used in the transfer process causes the embryos to wash back up the uterus into a Fallopian tube.

MULTIPLE BIRTHS In the general population, the chances of a multiple birth (twins or more) are about one in 80. IVF rates depend on the number of embryos transferred. Most programs try to transfer four to six embryos to increase the chances for one successful pregnancy. Such a transfer would pose a 20 percent chance of multiple births, with 1 to 3 percent of these resulting in triplets. Most IVF multiple births have been twins. One set of quadruplets has resulted from a four-embryo transfer.

Psychological and Emotional Dynamics of In Vitro Fertilization

► *What had gone wrong? What had I done? I felt like such a failure. Why had some of my fellow patients gotten pregnant with only one egg and not me? How could this have happened? After all, so many people were counting on me and praying for me.*

With the devastating news of this negative pregnancy test, I decided I was not going to lose this battle. To have a baby through IVF became the single greatest challenge of my life. On the next try, the medical team retrieved six ova and at least five were immature. For over two days we had no word about the progress of our "eggs." On the third day we were called for transfer. The medical team members were smiling from ear to ear. All six eggs had fertilized and would be transferred back into my uterus!

I cannot describe the exhilaration we experienced on hearing the news of a positive pregnancy test. Yet we had to remain cautious in spite of our joy. We still had nine long months ahead of us. In February we gave birth to an 8-lb., 5-oz. baby girl, the 47th in vitro baby to be born through the VIP program in Norfolk. And what a perfect gift she has been to us.

Dr. Linda Applegarth, a counseling psychologist, has graciously shared her IVF story in this chapter. Linda's infertility experience is indeed unique, and her courage, conviction, perseverance, and *luck* were rewarded with a beautiful baby daughter. *It is important to emphasize that luck plays a large role in every fertility treatment—especially IVF.* For every case like Linda's, eight or nine equally determined and courageous women will fail to get pregnant.

In addition to this high risk of disappointment, those who enter the IVF process also reexperience the old, familiar infertility feelings, intensified by the knowledge that this is the last medical resort.

► *There is so much waiting. There's the wait for the follicles to develop, the wait for ovulation and egg retrieval, the wait for fertilization and transfer, and the long, difficult wait until the pregnancy test.*

Much of IVF is waiting, watching, and hoping. The infertile couple is quite vulnerable and, in many respects, out of control again. From the first day of ovulation induction, the tension and anticipation build to an almost unbearable degree by the time embryo transfer occurs.

► *Ironically, there is a great deal of hope that's built into the IVF process, and all too often, the hope results in disappointment.*

From 80 to 90 percent of IVF patients have little difficulty reaching the transfer stage, only to be faced with a negative pregnancy test two weeks later. This can be a terrible letdown. One IVF specialist observed that many of his patients "feel pregnant" as soon as embryo transfer is done. When they learn the attempt was unsuccessful, they often experience the emotional aftermath of pregnancy loss. Where unsuccessful microsurgery is a gradual realization, an IVF failure is an immediate and devastating reality. Some patients who do get pregnant will miscarry shortly after.

► *Many husbands feel left out of the IVF process. Obviously their participation is crucial, but it is quite limited in comparison to their wives.*

The importance of the husband's support and caring is beyond measure. He often provides a much-needed reality factor and lends encouragement and optimism. Like infertility, however, the process inevitably takes its toll on the couple. After an unsuccessful try, the woman often worries that she didn't lie still long enough or in some other way rejected the embryo after transfer. The man is often depressed by the entire effort and concerned about his wife's reaction.

EMOTIONAL SUPPORT

► *I found it most beneficial to spend time with my fellow patients, but I also set aside time for myself—time for quiet and solitude.*

Many of the IVF medical team members share their patients' successes and failures. The doctor-patient relationship during IVF is one of intense, daily interaction for nearly two weeks as they work toward a common goal of pregnancy.

Nonetheless the medical team is *not* equipped to offer the emotional support that most patients need during this ordeal. In many IVF programs this vital function is taken on by the patients. Some have traveled far from home and miss the support of family and friends. Sharing joy and sadness with each other fills an important need. But patients can also become too close. Rumors and anxieties can spread like wildfire, and IVF often becomes an obsession to the exclusion of other activities and conversations. Ideally IVF programs will add professional counselors to their staffs.

SINGLE WOMEN

► *I feel extraordinarily lucky to be accepted into an IVF program in Northern California. Most programs will not accept single women.*

A single woman who wishes to undergo IVF may find the same problems encountered in the AID process (see Chapter 16). Many IVF programs will accept only a married couple. If she is accepted, a single woman may sense isolation and lack of support even more intensely than a couple.

Gamete Intrafallopian Tube Transfer (GIFT)

GIFT is a new medical technique recently reported by Ricardo Asch, M.D., a prominent Texas infertility specialist. GIFT is a similar procedure to IVF but has some important differences and advantages.

The Procedure

GIFT is a two-week process. Like IVF, superovulation is induced through fertility drugs. Daily monitoring is also conducted, one or more follicles are aspirated through laparoscopy, and the husband is asked to provide a fresh semen sample.

At this point, however, the process differs from IVF. With GIFT, the egg and sperm are not fertilized in the laboratory. Rather they are mixed together and injected by catheter into the Fallopian tube during a laparoscopy. Fertilization hopefully occurs in the tube and the embryo travels down to the uterus to implant. GIFT thus allows normal in vivo cell division to occur before implantation. Bed rest is usually recommended for one to two days following the laparoscopy.

In most cases GIFT is tried after one IVF attempt in which an ovum was fertilized to ensure that the egg can indeed be fertilized by the husband's sperm. It should also be noted that the GIFT procedure may fail to aspirate a mature ovum. In that case the ova may have to be incubated and IVF attempted.

Unfortunately GIFT is only available to women with at least one normal Fallopian tube. It may be an appropriate treatment for some types of male infertility and cervical mucus or sperm antibody problems. Most couples who undergo this procedure have unexplained infertility.

Cost

GIFT is somewhat less expensive than IVF because less laboratory work and resources are needed. The 1987 cost of GIFT was about $3500 per cycle. Part of this expense may be covered by some medical insurance carriers as part of infertility diagnosis. In the future GIFT may be performed during the diagnostic laparoscopy of the infertility workup if ovulation is occurring naturally.

Success Rates

GIFT offers about a 20 percent chance for success. A two- to three-cycle wait is recommended between attempts. For most couples a maximum of three or four tries is recommended.

Embryo Transfer

Embryo transfer is a medical technique that has been routinely used with cattle for years. Only recently has this technique been applied to human infertility. A "donor" fertile woman is artificially inseminated with sperm from an infertile woman's mate. The developing embryo is flushed from the donor's womb early in pregnancy and implanted in the infertile woman's uterus. This procedure is still experimental and has been tried in only a few clinics. Only a few live births have been reported so far.

Still embryo transfers may hold a promising future for infertile men and women. The method can be applied to several infertility situations. In cases of double infertility (both mates), both donor eggs and sperm can be used, and implanted in an infertile woman's uterus. A woman who is unable to carry a pregnancy can have her eggs extracted, fertilized with her husband's sperm, and implanted in a "donor's" womb.

Embryo transfer of eggs fertilized within the body is a nonsurgical technique and usually does not require hospitalization or anesthesia. It may be appropriate in cases where patients have declined further surgery, have surgically inaccessible ovaries, or have genetic reasons for avoiding a pregnancy using their own eggs.

CHAPTER 15

Diagnosis, Causes, and Treatment of Male Infertility

► *My wife's gynecologist phoned me and simply said, "You have no sperm. None." When I heard this news, I felt like someone had kicked me in the nuts.*

A male infertility problem is diagnosed in about 40 percent of couples seeking treatment. In another 10 percent of cases problems in both partners will contribute to their infertility. The incidence of male infertility may be increasing in our country. One study has suggested that there has been a decline in sperm count among American men over the past several decades. Although many urologists dispute the validity of this study, it is thought that the increasing incidence of sexually transmitted diseases, environmental pollutants, alcohol and drug abuse, exposure to X-rays or workplace toxins, and perhaps our modern, stressful life-style may be affecting male fertility.

Over the last 15 years, the field of andrology has evolved to study and treat disorders of the male reproductive system. Andrology is perhaps a generation behind gynecology in its research and understanding of physiology and reproduction. This is due both to a reluctance of many men to be tested and to prior assumptions by both society and the medical establishment that a couple's infertility was always caused by a problem in the female partner. Thus a discussion of the causes and treatments of male fertility problems is regrettably shorter than that of female infertility. With further research in andrology more infertile men may be treated successfully.

To facilitate understanding of the physiology and hormonal chemistry of the male reproductive system, which is discussed throughout this chapter, refer to "Human Reproduction," pages 93 to 103.

The Urologist

► *One of my patients was told by a number of internists that nothing could be done with his zero sperm count problem. I discovered he really didn't have a zero count. An X-ray revealed a cyst behind the prostate gland. Both ejaculatory ducts came into the cyst, which had no connection to the urethra. The whole system was dilated. The sperm were being produced and going into the cyst instead of the urethra. It was simple, under anesthesia, to go in through the urethra and make a slit in the floor of the prostate. His sperm count rose to 30 million a few months later.*

A urologist is a physician who specializes in disorders of the urinary system of both men and women. Some urologists are also andrologists and treat male reproductive problems. A physician with this specialized training is best qualified to interpret test results, prescribe treatment, or perform surgery for male infertility.

A urologist should be consulted when the semen analysis reports a low or zero sperm count or a problem with movement, shape, or volume of sperm, or when an abnormality such as obstruction, varicocele, or hormonal imbalance is suspected.

Optimally the couple and specialist work as a team, discussing tests, findings, and possible treatments as they progress through the workup. The couple should feel comfortable discussing their questions and concerns at any time. It is also strongly urged that they seek adequate emotional support.

Your gynecologist or infertility specialist may be able to refer you to a qualified urologist. Other sources of referral are RESOLVE, the American Fertility Society, or your local medical association.

The Male Infertility Workup

► *The semen analysis revealed a low count with no motility. A blood test showed a low level of testosterone. My initial reaction was shock. I felt my very masculinity was being challenged. All kinds of fears about my sexuality, losing my beard, even developing cancer filled my mind. Was my entire system out of whack? Finally I calmed down and began to ask questions: What does this mean? Can you fix the problem? Is surgery necessary?*

A man's initial appointment with a urologist is similar to that of a female infertility patient. The specialist will first meet the couple in his or her private office and take a detailed medical history of both partners. They will review any past surgeries (such as hernia repair) and exposure to drugs (including alcohol, cocaine, marijuana, and nicotine), current medications, occupational or environmental toxins, specific childhood illnesses (such as mumps), and past illnesses or diseases (such as viruses, infections, or sexually transmitted diseases). The specialist will ask about the frequency of intercourse and whether the couple has experienced any sexual problems.

Physical Examination

The history taking is followed by a thorough physical examination of the patient, including a careful examination of the penis, testes, prostate, and scrotum. The physician will check that each testicle is at least 1½ inches in length and will look for a varicocele, which can be felt in the scrotum while the patient is standing. They then meet again in the office to review the course of the workup and discuss physical findings, such as hernia or varicocele, and relevant medical history.

A Methodical Investigation

To ensure accuracy, the urologist repeats and personally interprets the semen analysis. It may provide some clue to the fertility problem. If not, the specialist and couple discuss and undergo other appropriate laboratory tests: biopsies, X-rays, surgeries, or fertility drugs. At the end of this workup both the physician and the couple should have more information and can work toward an appropriate resolution.

It is important to note that at least 10 percent of infertility is caused by problems in *both* partners. In fact the percentage of combined infertility problems may be higher, as some men with low sperm counts easily impregnate their mates, while others encounter years of fertility problems.

TABLE 15.1 Male Infertility Workup Tests

Procedure	Purpose	Benefits, Risks, and Inconveniences	Approximate Cost (1987)*
Initial Visit—interview, physical exam, routine lab work	To gather medical history of both partners, detect obvious anatomical or physical abnormalities which may be imparing fertility	May reveal causes of infertility without necessity of more costly, invasive testing	About $85 plus any lab work ordered
Semen Analysis	To evaluate number, motility and characteristics of sperm	Repeated analysis may be embarrassing, inconvenient and stressful	$50–75
Sperm Antibody Test	To test for antibodies to sperm in both partners	May give indications of fertility impairment in cases of long-term or unexplained infertility	$150
Testicular Biopsy	To determine whether low sperm count is caused by testicular or duct problem	Patient is exposed to risks of anesthesia and surgery	$240–300 for surgeon's fees plus $950 for anesthesiologist and hospital charges
Vasography	To evaluate structure of duct system and locate any obstructions	Patient is exposed to risks of anesthesia and surgery	$500 for radiologist, anesthesiologist and hospital charges
Fructose Test	To determine whether fructose from seminal vesicles is reaching the semen	An absence of fructose may suggest a congenital abnormality or absence of the seminal vesicles or vas deferens	$25; often included in the semen analysis charge
Hamster Egg Test	To provide informatin not available from semen analysis; assesses sperm's ability to penetrate a hamster ovum	Useful before costly IVF attempts. Cannot predict postively how sperm will interact with human egg	$250
Bovine Cervical Mucus Test	To determine sperm's ability to penetrate cervical mucus	May indicate possible motility problems or incompatibility of wife's mucus and husband's sperm.	$25–50

* Costs vary in different geographic areas. These charges are based on an average of the fees of several San Francisco area hospitals, specialists, and laboratories.

The Semen Analysis

► *The experience is just plain embarrassing. You are given a glass jar, sent to a bathroom (a totally asexual environment), and expected to produce a sample of semen—right now! If you can do it, you hand it to a nurse or technician, and they always seem to be females. The first couple of times they didn't even give me a bag or covering for the jar, so the entire waiting room audience could see it too! It seemed like everyone looked up from their magazines when I approached the desk. I also worried whether I'd pass the test: Were there enough sperm? Were they swimming fast enough?*

A semen analysis should be routinely performed at the onset of both the female and the male infertility workups. It is important to rule out any sperm abnormalities before extensive testing is done on the female partner. Because fevers or viruses can affect sperm count for months afterward, at least two collections should be done before a diagnosis of male infertility is confirmed.

Although the semen analysis is an important part of the workup, a single specimen may not be an accurate indicator of male fertility. Rather than relying on one test, most urologists prefer to obtain several semen analyses to observe the range of the patient's semen quality. Many personally perform the lab work on a fresh specimen obtained in their office.

COLLECTION PROCEDURE A precise collection procedure is essential to ensure accuracy and validity of the sample. The *entire* ejaculate should be collected in a clean, clear glass jar. In 90 percent of men, sperm are heavily concentrated in the first half of the ejaculate, so the second half is usually sperm poor. If the entire ejaculate is not collected, the count may be misleading.

The specimen should be collected at the laboratory or clinic where the analysis will be done. If this is not possible, it should be kept at room temperature and delivered to the lab within an hour of collection. At least 48 hours of abstinence is necessary before the test.

If religious beliefs prohibit masturbation, your specialist or clergy may have suggestions for obtaining a specimen without violating religious decrees. Some couples find it helpful to use a special condom to obtain the semen.

COUNTING AND EVALUATION After collection the ejaculate is drawn into a white blood cell pipette. It is diluted with a special solution that immobilizes the sperm and is placed in a blood cell counting chamber, which is divided into several large grids, each containing 16 smaller squares. The semen now has a volume one cell layer thick. Under the microscope, the number of sperm in five large grids are counted. This number is multipled by one million. The process is repeated with another set of five grids and the two numbers are averaged. This sperm count is obviously a rough estimate, with at least a 10 percent margin of error. For this reason semen analyses done by some general pathology labs are sometimes inaccurate or unreliable.

Sperm counts can vary considerably between men, and more importantly in the same man day to day. A sperm count of 20 million or more per cubic centimeter of semen, however, is usually considered normal (especially in the presence of good motility), although 60 to 100 million per cc are optimal counts.

Motility, or movement, of the sperm is also carefully observed within two hours of collection. Some scientists now believe that motility is more critical to male fertility than sperm count. A sperm cannot fertilize an egg unless it reaches the Fallopian tube and finds and penetrates the ovum.

To assess motility the percentage of moving sperm in ten random high-power microcopic fields is estimated. Ideally at least 60 percent of the sperm cells should be moving two to three hours after ejaculation. The quality of motility refers to the degree of forward progression, and is graded from zero (no movement) to four (excellent forward movement). Grades one and two are considered poor motility; while Grades three and four are rated good. Asthenospermia is a condition where less than half the sperm are motile.

The *morphology,* or shape and maturity, of the sperm cells are also examined. A smear of semen is placed on a slide, air-dried, and then stained. Approximately 100 cells are classified in six categories: (1) normal (oval) shape and maturity, (2) amorphous (irregular or immature shape and size), (3) tapered, (4) double-headed (or duplicate), (5) micro (too small), or (6) macro (too large). At least 60 percent of the sperm cells should be normal in shape, contour, and maturity.

Normally the semen is a liquid when ejaculated, coagulates quickly, and then reliquifies within 20 to 30 minutes. As part of the semen analysis the ejaculate is evaluated for its liquidity (*viscosity*). After ejaculation it should easily pour drop by drop.

The *volume* of the ejaculate varies among men, but about one teaspoonful is considered normal.

The *pH* of the semen is also tested. Normally it should register slightly alkaline, between 7.0 and 8.5 on the scale.

RESULTS OF THE SEMEN ANALYSIS The results of the semen test are generally categorized in one of four groups: (1) normal; (2) azoospermia (lack of any sperm); (3) abnormalities in several categories such as density, motility, morphology; or (4) isolated problems of one type (e.g., low sperm count).

The semen analysis should be repeated periodically during long-term infertility because acquired problems can reduce fertility during adulthood. These include hormonal imbalances, ejaculation abnormalities, exposure to drugs or toxic chemicals, and sperm antibodies.

TABLE 15.2 Semen Analysis Factors

Factor	Method	Evaluation Criteria	Reported Results
Sperm Count	Semen diluted and placed, one cell layer thick, in a counting chamber which is divided into grids	The number of sperm in five large grids is counted and multiplied by one million. A similar area is also counted and the two numbers averaged—a rough estimate with a 10 percent margin of error	A count of 20–100 million sperm per cc of ejaculate is reported "normal"; below 20 million is reported as "low sperm count"
Motility	Two to three hours after ejaculation, the percentage of moving sperm in 10 random high power microscopic fields is estimated	Degree of forward progression is rated on a scale of 0–4 (none–excellent)	Grades One and Two are reported as "poor motility"; Grades Three and Four as "good motility"
Morphology	A smear of semen is air dried on a slide and under the microscope 100 cells are studied for shape and maturity	Sperm cells are categorized: (1) normal (mature with oval shape); (2) amorphous (immature shape or size); (3) tapered; (4) doubleheaded; (5) micro (too small); (6) macro (too big)	If 60 percent or more of the cells fall into Category 1, a "normal morphology" result is reported. Less than 60 percent indicates abnormal sperm morphology
Viscosity	The liquidity of the sperm 20–30 minutes after ejaculation	Should pour easily drop by drop	If semen remains gelled, poor viscosity is reported
Volume	Measuring the amount of semen which is ejaculated	2–5 cc is considered within normal range	Less than 2cc is considered low volume; greater than 5 cc is considered excessive volume
pH	Ejaculate is chemically tested for pH	Normal range is slightly alkaline—7.0 to 8.5	Any variation of this range would be reported as abnormal pH—either too acidic or excessively alkaline

Sperm Antibody Test

A male workup may also involve a test for antibodies to sperm in both partners. Like viruses and bacteria, sperm are a foreign substance and have the potential to engage the body's immune system.

A small percentage of women have antibodies to sperm similar to the immunity developed to a particular disease. The antibodies occur in vaginal or cervical secretions and kill the sperm or cause them to clump together. Men may also develop antibodies to their own sperm, especially after a vasectomy is done.

Indications for sperm antibody testing include a normal sperm count with poor motility, clumping of sperm, a poor postcoital test result, a good count with poor motility after a vasectomy reversal, and unexplained infertility.

A number of laboratory tests can be performed to check for the presence of sperm antibodies in either partner. (See Chapter 12 for further discussion of sperm antibody testing and treatment.)

Hormonal Blood Tests

In most men, the levels of FSH, LH, and testosterone fluctuate hourly. However, blood tests that reveal unusually high or low hormonal levels may indicate endocrinological or testicular problems that merit further investigation.

Testicular Biopsy

If the semen analysis shows a very low count or no sperm at all and hormonal levels are normal, a biopsy can be performed to determine whether the problem is caused by a blockage or impaired sperm production. A tissue sample is taken from the testicle in an outpatient procedure under general or local anesthesia. Although this is a simple procedure, the surgeon must handle the tissue carefully. It is easily destroyed and must be preserved in a special solution. The tissue is examined under the microscope for the presence of sperm-generating cells. Absence of these cells indicates a testicular problem and, sadly, permanent infertility. If the sperm cells are present, the urologist can then investigate obstruction problems.

Vasography

Vasography is a test that checks the structure of the duct system and locates any obstructions. Defining these areas in advance increases the chances of successful microsurgery. During this procedure the scrotum is opened under anesthesia, a dye is injected into the duct system, and X-rays are taken to reveal any blockages.

Fructose Test

When working properly the seminal vesicles add fructose to the semen. A negative fructose test suggests a congenital absence of the vas deferens or seminal vesicles.

Hamster Egg Test (Sperm Penetration Assay)

The hamster egg test assesses the capacity of the sperm to penetrate a hamster ovum, a quality not measured by the standard semen analysis. The gelatinous zone surrounding the egg is removed, and the sperm are prepared in the lab and placed adjacent to the egg to attempt penetration. If the sperm have less than a 10 percent penetration score, a male fertility problem is suspected.

Before a couple undergoes the expense and stress of in vitro fertilization, the hamster egg test is often used to confirm the sperm's ability to fertilize. It may also reveal male fertility problems in cases of unexplained infertility; in cases of varicocele the test can help physician and patient decide whether surgery is indicated.

This test, however, cannot assess the sperm's motility or predict how the sperm will react to the zona pellucida (outer covering) of a human egg.

Bovine Cervical Mucus Test

This test checks the sperm's ability to penetrate cervical mucus. Cervical mucus from cows is used because it closely resembles human mucus and is easily handled in the laboratory. The mucus is drawn into a capillary pipette (a long glass tube) and inserted in a sample of semen. The progress of the sperm is observed for an hour and a half. A motility problem is suspected if the sperm cannot travel a determined distance through the mucus. In such cases intrauterine insemination (IUI) may be indicated.

Diagnostic Categories of Male Infertility and Their Treatment

For decades low sperm count was blamed for all male fertility problems. There is now increasing evidence that other factors can also contribute to male infertility. Unfortunately there is little knowledge of how such problems affect male fertility. More research is needed on the subjects of immunology, sperm production and motility, infection, and characteristics of seminal fluid.

Low Sperm Counts/Poor Motility

Fevers, illnesses, and infections can temporarily affect sperm count for up to three months. Before a low sperm count is diagnosed, two or more semen analyses should be performed over at least three months. Sperm motility can be affected by a varicocele, prolonged periods of abstinence from ejaculation, and exposure to heat from saunas or hot tubs.

Problems with persistent low sperm count (oligospermia) or poor motility do account for more than half of male infertility complaints. A low sperm count usually refers to less than 20 million sperm per cubic centimeter of ejaculate. Poor motility is diagnosed when half or more of the sperm are not swimming properly.

In half or more of these cases the cause of the problem is unknown. This condition is termed "idiopathic oligospermia." In other instances low sperm counts may be caused by varicocele, duct obstruction, undescended testicles, retrograde ejaculation, environmental or workplace toxins, surgery, drug use, hormonal imbalances, some medications (especially cancer treatments), in utero exposure to DES, or neurological disorders.

Treating a low sperm count problem is a difficult task. There is no known "cure" because the abnormality itself is not fully understood. In fact about 25 percent of couples with this problem will conceive with no treatment at all! Good motility and an especially fertile female partner improve the odds for a pregnancy.

IN VITRO FERTILIZATION (IVF) OR GAMETE INTRAFALLOPIAN TUBE TRANSFER (GIFT)
Initially these options were offered only to couples whose infertility was caused by tubal or other problems in the female partner. They are now sometimes offered to couples with a wide range of fertility complaints, including low sperm count.

SPLIT EJACULATE In cases of low sperm count, some urologists will recommend IUI with a split ejaculate. During this procedure, the semen is concentrated in a fraction of the original volume and then artificially inseminated into the wife's uterus. Success rates for IUI run betwen 25 and 30 percent.

BLUE ICE AND BOXER SHORTS Some urologists recommend "blue ice" treatment to lower testicular temperature. Blue ice is actually a combination of water and a few household chemicals; it is packaged in plastic containers and sold in many stores. After the packet is frozen, it is wrapped in a towel and placed near the scrotum overnight. There has been some success reported with this method.

Other urologists believe that wearing close-fitting underwear, which hold the scrotum close to the body, may increase testicular temperature.

They recommend switching to boxer shorts to lower the temperature and hopefully elevate sperm count. This theory is somewhat refuted by the several generations of American men who wore close-fitting underwear and still fathered many children.

FERTILITY DRUG TREATMENT Use of fertility drugs probably offers only about the same chances for success as the spontaneous pregnancy rate (25 percent) achieved with no treatment at all. Individual successes, of course, depend on both luck and other fertility factors in both partners. In many instances success rates are much lower. Most couples conclude that drug therapy is not worth the stress and bother. On the other hand a few couples opt for fertility drugs because they have been trying unsuccessfully for a pregnancy for years and feel they have no chance for a biological child without treatment.

The FDA has approved the experimental use of some fertility drugs for males. This means that the drugs are not available for routine clinical use but are prescribed by a specialist to study and test their value and the patient must give his informed consent. It is hoped that these drugs will increase sperm count through chemical stimulation of the pituitary, testes, or hypothalamus.

The drug treatments described below will sometimes increase the sperm count to 20 million or more, which some patients consider tremendous increases. Unfortunately, since the technique for counting sperm is inexact, changes of a few million are usually not significant.

At this time the drugs used to treat specific types of male infertility are: clomiphene, HCG (human chorionic gonadotropin), HMG (human menopausal gonadotropin), bromocriptine, and testosterone. Each has specific uses and indications (see Chapter 9 for further discussion):

- *Clomiphene* is a synthetic estrogen commonly prescribed for ovulation induction. In the male it blocks the testosterone receptor site in the hypothalamus, which results in secretion of GnRH, LH, and FSH. The LH prompts the Leydig cells in the testicle to increase testosterone production, and the FSH stimulates the production and maturation of germ cells. Sperm counts then increase.

  Low dosages of clomiphene are usually prescribed for several months. A common therapy is 25 mg for 25 days, followed by a five-day rest, after which the sequence is repeated. Hormonal levels are usually checked after two months, and treatment may be continued for as long as a year if hormone levels remain normal.

  Side effects vary among men but can include blurred vision, and slight enlargement or tenderness of the breasts. Liver damage is a rare side effect. When taking clomiphene, exercise caution while driving or performing chores that require alertness.

There is a 50 percent chance for improvement in sperm count and motility. Some studies claim a 20 percent or even greater pregnancy rate after male clomiphene therapy, depending on whether other fertility problems are present in either partner.

- *HCG and HMG* The hormone HCG has been used to treat undescended testicle problems for several decades. Recently it has also been prescribed in some cases of low sperm count. In cases of abnormal hypothalamic activity HMG (Pergonal) may also be prescribed with HCG.

  There isn't much scientific evidence that either drug is effective for improving sperm count, unless there is a specific hormonal imbalance. These drugs should be considered only in cases of long-term, repeatedly low sperm counts. The drugs are administered by injection in carefully monitored and adjusted doses.

  The side effects may include temporary breast enlargement and weight gain. The drugs are expensive, and no advantage has been shown in using them instead of clomiphene when no hormone problem exists.

  The use of HCG alone or with HMG improves sperm count in 50 percent of idiopathic oligospermia cases. The pregnancy rate, however, is only about 20 percent. In cases of significant hormonal imbalance, HCG and/or HMG produce higher pregnancy rates.

- *Bromocriptine* The role of prolactin hormone in the male is not fully understood. In rare cases, however, some men develop elevated prolactin levels and bromocriptine (Parlodel) may be prescribed. To date there is little data on success rates.

- *Testosterone* When other hormonal treatments fail, some urologists may prescribe testosterone. It is given for a short time and then stopped in the hope that a rebound effect will occur: Sperm production will be abruptly halted and then quickly resume. Because some patients experience a permanent cessation of sperm production, this is a controversial treatment not recommended by all specialists. There are reports, however, of 20 to 40 percent success rates in improving sperm count.

Varicocele

A varicocele is a varicose vein of the scrotum. Between 10 and 15 percent of all men have a detectable varicocele, but it affects fertility in only about half the cases. It is also thought that some men may have a varicocele that cannot be clinically diagnosed.

A varicocele forms when the valves of the vein fail to close behind the retreating blood. The blood backs up and pools, and the vein swells. Varicoceles nearly always occur on the left side, near the epididymis. The blood travels through the renal vein and empties into the vena cava at an angle on the left side; the right side empties directly into the vena cava. The angle encountered on the left side causes more opportunities for dysfunction.

EFFECT ON FERTILITY In about 25 percent of infertile men, varicoceles cause variable sperm count, motility, and morphology problems. They are the most easily identifiable cause of male infertility, ranging from large (visible through scrotal skin), to moderate (easily palpable), to small (difficult to detect). There is no relationship, however, between the size of the varicocele and the sperm count.

It is not known exactly how a varicocele reduces sperm count, although one popular theory suggests that the accumulated blood in the vein increases scrotal temperature and slows sperm production.

There are two clues that the varicocele is actively reducing fertility. The first is atrophy of the testicle, usually on the same side as the varicocele. The second is a stress pattern detected in the semen analysis, where increased numbers of tapered and/or immature sperm heads are observed.

TREATMENTS Varicoceles can be treated with either surgery or a radiological procedure.

A quick and fairly simple operation can be performed under general or local anesthesia. An incision is made in the lower abdomen, and the internal spermatic vein is tied off rather than removed. This method prevents the backflow of blood into the scrotum. Many urologists now perform this surgery on an outpatient basis, and normal activity can be resumed in several weeks. (See Chapters 5 and 8 for a discussion of surgery.) Sperm count improves in about 75 percent of cases, although this percentage varies between individuals depending on their count before surgery. The pregnancy rate is 40 to 50 percent after surgery if no other fertility problems are present. If surgery is not successful, drug therapy may be tried with either clomiphene or HCG.

The radiological technique is a fairly new, nonsurgical treatment and has not been extensively tested. The radiologist inserts a small catheter into the femoral vein in the groin, guides it through the interior vena cava and down into the spermatic vein, and places a detachable balloon or coil in this area to block the flow of blood. This method should be performed by an experienced radiologist trained in the technique. The cost of the procedure is about the same as for varicocele surgery. Studies are now being published about the technique and reported success rates are close to those for varicocele surgery. The patient is exposed to radiation, however, and the physician does not have the direct view of the varicocele that would be possible in surgery. This procedure may be more appropriate for men who have a recurrent varicocele problem that has not responded to surgical treatment.

Duct Obstruction

A small number of men with persistently low sperm counts (10 million or less) have an obstruction that inhibits the sperm's journey to the urethra. A zero sperm count may also suggest an obstruction if a testicular biopsy has ruled out problems with sperm production. Diagnosis is made through testicular biopsy, X-rays, or surgical exploration of the scrotum under anesthesia. During surgery an incision is usually made into the epididymis to locate the sperm.

Obstructions, which most commonly occur in the epididymis, may be caused by congenital problems, infections, or traumas to the scrotum. Congenital problems can include epididymal scarring or an absence of part of the vas deferens. In utero DES exposure can also cause anatomical abnormalities of the testicles or duct system. Infection, particularly from sexually transmitted diseases, can cause scarring of the epididymis. Secondary damage following an initial infection can also occur in other areas of the duct system. Dysfunction of the epididymis can be caused by a complete or partial obstruction or by inflammation (epididymitis).

TREATMENT If the male evaluation, including the biopsy, shows that an obstruction is present, surgery is indicated. If the biopsy results are not definitive, drug treatment to elevate sperm count may be recommended.

Surgery is performed under general anesthesia, usually on an outpatient basis. A scrotal exploration is done to locate, and hopefully bypass, the obstruction. As with varicocele surgery, limited activity is required for several weeks.

Ejaculation Abnormalities

A small percentage of infertile men have a problem either with the volume or viscosity of their ejaculate, or with an absence of semen. Retrograde ejaculation, a condition where the sperm spill out of the urethra into the bladder, can occur as a result of previous surgery or nerve damage caused by diabetes, or for no apparent reason.

EXCESSIVE EJACULATE In most cases ejaculation problems involve an excessive amount of semen. This dilutes the sperm concentration in the seminal fluid. There may not be a great enough concentration of sperm to form the phalanxes necessary to penetrate the cervical mucus.

Treatment is sometimes attempted with the split ejaculate method, in which the sperm are concentrated in less semen and artificially inseminated.

TOO LITTLE EJACULATE Too small an amount of ejaculate may indicate a blockage in the seminal vesicles, which contribute fructose sugar and most of the seminal fluid. A simple laboratory test can check the semen for the presence of fructose. An absence of this sugar suggests a blockage in the seminal vesicles.

VISCOSITY PROBLEMS Ideally enzymes produced by the seminal vesicles coagulate the semen shortly after ejaculation. Other enzymes produced by the prostate gland cause it to reliquify 5 to 20 minutes later.

Sometimes the ejaculate remains coagulated and does not reliquify. In some cases the sperm may be trapped within the coagulated ejaculate and unable to swim through the cervical mucus.

TREATMENT Several methods can be tried: the split ejaculate method described above; cocoa butter vaginal suppositories to liquify the semen; or an experimental approach that adds an enzyme produced by the salivary glands to the ejaculate before it is inseminated. This last remedy was discovered by a urologist in the Midwest who, frustrated with an ejaculate that would not liquify, spit into it. To his amazement it liquified! If the postcoital test reveals good cervical mucus with a low sperm count in the volume, intrauterine insemination may be tried to maximize chances for pregnancy. Unfortunately, none of these treatments are very successful in improving pregnancy rates.

Endocrinological Abnormalities

► *Several of my hormonal levels are quite low. We eventually traced this to a congenital problem with my testicles. For years I didn't know about it, and I actually found a bit of humor in this ignorance. I thought back to fumbling around in the dark for prophalytics. The humor took a bit of the pain away.*

Hormonal abnormalities occur in less than 5 percent of infertile men and may result in low or even zero sperm counts. These imbalances are sometimes caused by head trauma, pituitary tumors, infection, drug use, chemotherapy, or Klinefelter's syndrome (a hereditary condition that causes a complete absence of sperm).

In most cases, however, the imbalance is caused by reduced function of the pituitary gland. These are the cases in which fertility drug treatment is often effective.

DES

Unfortunately there have not been as many studies of DES sons as of DES daughters, and little medical information is available. It is known that DES sons may develop anatomical abnormalities, such as epididymal cysts or smaller testicles, or have problems with low sperm counts.

DES sons should inform physicians of their exposure, and those who suspect reproductive problems should seek the advice of a urologist knowledgeable about DES effects on males. DES Action USA is also a good resource for readings, referrals, and emotional support (see Chapter 10 and Appendix A.)

Vasectomy Reversal

► *I got married when I was 22 years old. My wife and I promptly had two boys in four years. We were happy, didn't want to have any more kids, and figured we'd be married forever. I had a vasectomy to simplify birth control.*

Our marriage fell apart about five years later. We shared custody of the boys and I had no interest in marrying again until I met Tina. We were both in our midthirties when we decided to get married.

This is Tina's first marriage and having a child was very important to her. Although my sons were 10 and 12, I decided I'd also like to have another child.

Since it was ten years since my vasectomy, the specialist warned me that a reversal might not be successful. Even if it was, it could take years for the sperm count to rise high enough to get Tina pregnant. I wanted to try anyhow.

The reversal was done under a local anesthetic, so I was conscious but pretty groggy. The doctors told me this was a better route to go than general anesthesia, only I had to promise not to move! No problem: There was no way I was going to move during that surgery!

I was pretty sore for about a week. My sperm count rose steadily over the next six months. About a year later Tina got pregnant, and my third son was born nine months later.

Every year about 500,000 American men who believe they have finished fathering babies elect to be sterilized by vasectomy. This simple surgical procedure, performed under local anesthesia in the doctor's office, severs the vas deferens. This prevents any sperm from reaching the urethra. Sex drive, performance, and quantity of seminal fluid are not affected.

Each year several thousand of these men regret their decision. They may divorce and remarry or tragically lose one or more of their children. In any case they consider restoring their fertility through vasectomy reversal.

The Surgery

The surgery is performed under general, spinal, or local anesthesia (see Chapter 5 for a discussion of surgery and anesthesia). Fine microsurgery techniques are used to realign the severed vas exactly. This is painstaking work as the inner canal of the vas is only about 1/64 inch in diameter. The ends are carefully sutured with a microscopic material only three times as thick as a red blood cell. Vasectomy reversals are often done on an outpatient basis. Soreness usually persists for a week or so.

Success Rates

Vasectomy reversals are most successful if done within ten years of the original sterilization. The vasectomy can cause pressure to build within the epididymis, which may rupture the duct. The longer the duct is under this pressure, the greater the chances of rupture. It is, of course, possible that epididymal damage can be repaired through microsurgery.

If the reversal is done within ten years, normal sperm count is restored in 80 percent of patients within a year, and the pregnancy rate is about 60 percent. The incidence of birth defects or other abnormalities in children fathered after vasectomy reversal is no greater than in the general population.

Psychological and Emotional Impact of Male Infertility

► *My sperm count was very low, and the sperm were immature—without tails. For some reason, my testicles didn't mature and my testosterone level is low. It was quite a shock to find this out. Although I was grateful that my equipment worked, I also worried whether I would be more susceptible to cancer. The doctor evaluated my beard and voice, and suggested hormone shots. I felt almost embarrassed. I wondered if I was smaller than other men. Did I last as long or ejaculate as much?*

Infertility raises many intense emotional and psychological issues for us both as individuals and as couples. Part One examines many of these dynamics in detail. A few issues unique to male infertility are briefly discussed in this section.

Anger and grief, commonly experienced with any fertility problem, are focused on the husband. The wife often feels angry and sad that she cannot conceive her mate's child. She may feel he has let her down in one of the most important ways she can imagine. She may also feel it is unacceptable to express these strong, conflicting emotions to her partner. The husband is trying to cope with a gamut of feelings: fear that he has disappointed his wife, inadequacy, and grief for the loss of a biological child. This is a devastating experience for both partners and requires time to absorb and grieve.

Public Reaction

A low sperm count or male fertility surgery often results in the couple's "going public" about the man's problem. Although relatives and friends may still ask his wife about the treatment and prognosis, he may now be ridiculed for his inadequacy.

Many people also associate male infertility with impotence. While listening to their friends' cruel jokes, many infertile men secretly worry either that they will lose their masculinity and sexual potency or that others will think they have.

Cultural Conditioning

From a young age many American males are taught to hide their feelings and, above all, not to acknowledge or express pain. When infertility is diagnosed, many men revert to these patterns and refuse to discuss their reactions or grief.

Our society reinforces this behavior. Most of the couple's friends and relatives will assume the woman has the medical problem. She, rather than he, will be asked why they are childfree and offered endless advice. With his wife fielding the questions and comments, the man can further recede into his isolation.

A man may also react differently to an infertility problem than his wife. Earlier we suggested that women usually grieve longer and more deeply over fertility loss, mainly because many are taught to define their identity through their relationships (e.g., wife and mother) rather than an occupation or career. Men, on the other hand, generally derive more status and identity through career status. One urologist observed:

► *Many of my patients treat their infertility with the same rational, businesslike approach that they would use on the job. They want to define the problem, consider their options, make a decision, and move on.*

Although his problem is painful, an infertile man may channel his frustration and anger into his work. He must, however, confront the loss of his biological offspring.

Ethnic Heritage

► *I have had patients from the Middle East and Africa who have been completely devastated by their fertility problem and have told me they would consider suicide if they could not father a child.*

America is a mixture of diverse subcultures and ethnic traditions. Some of these heritages place an extraordinary emphasis on fertility and siring children. Just as some women from different ethnic backgrounds feel especially inadequate when told of their infertility, many men from a variety of "macho" backgrounds may feel inferior, demasculinized, or worthless.

It is often difficult for these men to ask for or receive emotional support from their peers or family. Even worse, many of these cultures also attach a stigma to seeking professional counseling or therapy. Fortunately there is support available to all infertile men and women from RESOLVE and other support organizations (see Appendix A).

CHAPTER 16

Artificial Insemination

► *Because we had a combination of fertility problems, our specialist suggested we try inseminating my husband's sperm directly into my uterus. Although we were glad there was a treatment that might work, we were also reminded that we couldn't get pregnant the "normal" way.*

► *After I learned I was sterile, I was angry and bitter for months. I wouldn't discuss it with my wife and didn't want her talking to anyone else about it.*

After a while, though, I began to consider AID. I finally convinced Nina I was serious. From my perspective, the child would be half ours and we could control the pregnancy. Because I was the advocate, I felt powerful rather than useless.

Artificial insemination is the process by which sperm are inserted by syringe into the vagina or uterus. There are two types: AIH (*a*rtificial *i*nsemination by *h*usband's sperm) and AID (*a*rtificial *i*nsemination by *d*onor's sperm).

Artificial Insemination by Husband's Sperm (AIH)

AIH is usually used to bypass cervical mucus that is inhospitable to sperm. Specialists disagree about whether it increases fertility in cases of low sperm count, poor motility, or sperm antibodies.

The sperm are usually washed, by repeated centrifuging, from the protein and chemicals of the ejaculate before the insemination. Only a small amount of semen-free sperm are then inseminated into the uterus through a small plastic tube. Sperm washing reduces but does not eliminate the small risk of allergic reaction, shock, or infection from this procedure.

Using the husband's sperm for artificial insemination raises no psychological, moral, ethical, or legal questions. If the semen is inseminated directly into the uterus (intrauterine insemination or IUI), success rates range from 10–25 percent. Only about 13 percent of AIH attempts result in pregnancy if the semen is inseminated into the vagina. The latter procedure is often done only as a last resort, after other male and female fertility treatments have failed.

Artificial Insemination by Donor (AID)

The AID procedure, which inseminates donor sperm into a fertile woman, has been a commonly used treatment for male infertility for over 40 years. About 5 percent of couples encountering male infertility will try AID, and between 15,000 and 20,000 babies are conceived annually in the United States by this process.

AID has always been and remains a controversial social and legal issue. Many in our society disapprove of the practice, and couples undergoing AID often do not tell friends or family about their treatment. The laws regarding AID vary from one state to another. Several states have adopted some form of Section V of the Uniform Paternity Act, which deals exclusively with AID. In these states a husband consenting to an AID pregnancy is considered the legal father. Other states address the paternity issue via other statutes or court decisions. In a few states the law is vague or silent about paternity in AID offspring. Questions of child support, for example, may remain at issue. If you are considering AID, be sure to seek expert legal advice from an attorney familiar with the laws of your state.

Despite its controversy, AID can be a joyous, life-affirming process. For thousands of infertile couples who cannot be medically treated and for single women who desire a child, it creates a path to pregnancy and parenting. One prominent infertility specialist who has facilitated and monitored over 400 artificial insemination pregnancies considers AID "the happiest, most positive part of my infertility practice."

Deciding on AID

► *The decision was easy for us. My husband was sterile and we wanted kids. He wasn't worried about the other man's sperm. He said, "If it grows within you, it's part of me."*

► *I preferred adoption to AID. I felt I couldn't participate in AID at all, and that gave me feelings of impotency.*

Initially all couples must confront the painful reality of their infertility. These emotions are discussed in Chapters 1, 2, and 15. After sorting through and resolving their feelings, they have the strength and perspective to consider treatment options, including AID.

IS AID RIGHT FOR US? Many factors enter into a couple's decision to pursue AID. First they must believe that it is unlikely the wife will get pregnant by her husband. This is a logical conclusion if the husband has a zero sperm count or a congenital absence of the vas deferens. Nature has prevented fertility in these instances. However, a low sperm count or poor motility is involved in most cases of male infertility. The husband is not clinically sterile and there is a chance he can father a child. If the couple does accept the unlikelihood of pregnancy with the husband's sperm, they must decide whether they are both comfortable with the wife being impregnated with another man's sperm. This is a tough question for both and may take some time to answer.

Next they must balance the pros and cons of an AID pregnancy. The advantages are: the wife will experience pregnancy and birth; the couple can ensure that the baby has good prenatal care and nutrition; the child will carry his or her mother's genes; and the couple can have a baby without the red tape and waiting involved with agency or private adoptions. On the other hand AID poses a number of unique challenges to the family, such as legal and moral considerations and search issues for the child (further explored at the end of this chapter.) To facilitate decision making, many couples study literature about AID, speak with health care professionals, and seek private or infertility support group counseling.

BEING IN ACCORD AS A COUPLE

► *I had a hard time believing Jim wouldn't mind the AID. It took quite a while for him to convince me and for both of us to agree that AID was the right option.*

Although being in agreement about AID is crucial, few couples initially agree on this option. In fact the wife often pushes for AID treatment soon after her husband learns he is infertile. She wants a biological child, and this is a way to get pregnant. At first her husband is usually less comfortable with this option; AID won't give *him* a biological child.

Pursuing AID while in conflict is not advisable; after the fact is *not* the time to decide AID was the wrong decision. It takes time, honest and open communication, and patience to reach a mutual decision. Physicians and counselors find that couples who have spent months of careful consideration do best with this process.

Entering the AID process after careful thought can also strengthen the couple's relationship. Bonina Cohen, a northern California counselor, studied the psychological aspects of the process, as well as the differences between AIH and AID couples. She reports that although most AID couples found the process quite stressful, they expressed greater marital satisfaction and less instability than a sample of fertile couples. Those who conceived with AID responded they were happy to experience pregnancy, relieved they were past infertility, and glad they sought counseling. Couples who were unsuccessful in achieving pregnancy reported they were still happy they had confronted the problem.

Donor Sperm

► *I eyed every man in the building, wondering if he might be the donor. I later found out that the specimens are brought by a middleman; the donor never comes to the clinic.*

The couple who has opted for AID is naturally concerned about the health, identity, and physical and mental characteristics of the donor. In most cases donors are students (commonly medical students in metropolitan areas) and are chosen differently in each AID program. Their motives are usually a mixture of altruism, ego gratification, and financial reward.

Matching can be done for general physical characteristics such as race and hair and eye coloring, but the child may still have very different physiological characteristics from the husband. For example, blood can be matched for a general type such as O, but there are now 50 characteristics for which blood is typed. A detailed typing later in the child's life may reveal significant differences from the husband's blood. This can cause fear and confusion if he or she is unaware of the donor.

There may be a waiting list for non-Caucasian donors. Black and Asian donors are in much more demand either because of a scarcity of these ethnic groups in medical schools or because of their unwillingness to donate sperm. There is usually no wait for Caucasian donors.

SCREENING DONORS Depending on the physician or AID program, donor screening can vary from the meticulous to the nonexistent. Researchers at the University of Wisconsin, for example, surveyed 400 physicians performing AID and found that only 12 percent performed chromosome tests on the donors, and only 30 percent tested for traits that would indicate hereditary factors.

In light of the recent epidemic of acquired immune deficiency syndrome (AIDS or HTLV-III/LAV virus), most experts now recommend thorough screening of the donor and his sperm for the presence of AIDS and other sexually transmitted diseases, such as gonorrhea, herpes, mycoplasma (ureaplasma), chlamydia, syphilis, and hepatitis B, as well as Tay Sachs disease, sickle cell anemia, and other pathogens. When considering an AID program, inquire how donors are selected and what information is available about them. Some physicians allow the couple to select the donor from files that usually contain a serial number and very general physical characteristics. Other specialists select the donors themselves, after an extensive interview with the couple. In all cases donor anonymity is preserved.

Initially a thorough medical questionnaire should be filled out by the donor, directed specifically toward inherited health characteristics, past incidence or exposure to disease, and number and sex of previous sexual partners. Some physicians and clinics only use donors they know personally.

In a recent article in *The New England Journal of Medicine,* Drs. Laurene Mascola and Mary Guinan advise that donors be tested for AIDS and other sexually transmitted and genetic diseases at the time of collection. They recommend freezing the sample and, if initial testing is negative, retesting the donor three to six months later. If testing is again negative at that time, the frozen sample can then be inseminated. Although success rates with frozen sperm are lower than those of fresh, many experts feel that using frozen sperm is necessary, in order to rule out the chance transmitting a serious or even fatal disease through insemination.

If you are considering AID treatment, discuss the issues of donor screening and fresh or frozen sperm use with your specialist.

SPERM BANKS There are now a number of clinics and laboratories, sometimes called sperm banks, that store and dispense donor sperm. Fresh sperm may be available, as well as frozen sperm, which is stored in ampules, or tiny straws, in liquid nitrogen at –324°F for five to ten years. The quality control of these banks varies, so the consumer must choose carefully.

There is now a sperm bank that invites men of superior intelligence to become donors. To qualify as a recipient, a couple must be married and the wife must have a certain IQ level. This bank has been criticized for having a "master race" motivation.

Bills have been introduced in many state legislatures to regulate all sperm banks. Efforts are also being made to limit the multiple use of a single donor's sperm (the American Fertility Society recommends a maximum of 15 pregnancies per donor). In one instance researchers found one donor responsible for 50 pregnancies. There has also been some concern about the potential for unknowing incest among AID offspring, particularly in small communities where donors may be scarce. The odds, however, of the children of the same donor meeting and deciding to marry are very slight.

The Medical Procedure

► *When I saw the syringe, I almost jumped off the table in last minute panic. But, once again, my desire for a child kept me in place and I watched the "stranger's" semen enter my body. The procedure itself is not painful, but the emotional turmoil is quite strong.*

► *At first I viewed AID almost as a rapelike act, perhaps because once again I was not in control of the situation. But by the time I started the inseminations, it felt like just another medical procedure.*

AID, a relatively simple medical procedure, is usually done in a doctor's office. Insemination is generally tried two days a month, timed to coincide as closely as possible with ovulation. Although some physicians use sonograms or hormonal blood tests to pinpoint ovulation, others rely solely on the BBT chart. As the above quotes illustrate, women's reactions to the medical procedure of insemination vary considerably.

During the insemination procedure the woman lies on the examination table and a speculum is inserted into her vagina. Using a syringe, either the physician or her husband then deposits donor sperm at the cervical opening. At the couple's request, most specialists will allow the husband to perform the insemination. This gesture includes the husband in the process and may ease his feelings of inadequacy or isolation.

The woman then rests on the table for 15 to 30 minutes to give the sperm time to reach the Fallopian tubes. A sponge or insemination cap designed to fit over the cervix may be used to prolong the sperm's contact with that area. Sometimes a tampon is placed in back of the cap, although this technique does not seem to affect the success rate. Some women experience slight cramping after the procedure.

The couple may be advised to avoid intercourse on insemination days as the husband's semen may be deleterious to the donor sperm. Most clinics, if requested, will mix small amounts of the husband's sperm with the donor's for psychological reasons. In such cases there is a possibility, however slight, that the child may be fathered by the husband. Some husbands also feel that in this way they are at least symbolically participating in the conception of the child.

Success Rates

Overall success rates run between 40 and 80 percent and conception is usually achieved within six months of the first treatment. Using frozen sperm, rather than fresh, may decrease the chances for success by 10 to 15 percent. About 60 percent of couples get pregnant within the first six months through AID; another 10 to 15 percent achieve pregnancy by the end of one year. The ratio of male infants born is 55 to 45, probably due to the timing of insemination. If the fertility drug clomiphene has been used to stimulate ovulation, this ratio changes to an even 50/50 chance for a boy or girl.

AID is usually tried with a healthy woman who has no known fertility problem. It is traumatic and expensive to investigate female infertility if there is no reason to suspect it. However, if pregnancy does not occur after six tries, the physician will usually recommend a female infertility workup. Attempts to inseminate are usually halted after a year, although the couple may determine how long to continue treatment.

It is not unusual for the stress of AID to cause irregular cycles for the first few months. This usually corrects itself. Fertility drugs are not used unless indicated by an ovulatory problem. In fact there is evidence that women are *less* fertile with drugs than without if no ovulatory problem exists.

Psychological Reactions to the AID Process

Although AID is a fairly routine medical procedure, it is a complex psychological and emotional experience. Couples undergoing periodic inseminations commonly experience a number of reactions.

ISOLATION

► *We felt estranged from even other infertiles. We were "in the closet" and missed the recognition and sympathy they were getting.*

During the AID process, a couple may feel an even greater isolation than with other types of infertility. Because most people are critical and unable to understand their struggle, many couples do not tell anyone they are involved in AID. Few AID programs require counseling, and many physicians find it difficult to deal with their patients' emotional reactions.

Some couples cope with this estrangement by telling a few trusted friends and relatives. Others join an AID support group and discuss their feelings only with those experiencing the same issues. Often couples find it an enormous relief to share their situation and cannot stop talking at such meetings.

If a group situation is not comfortable for you, consider private infertility counseling or meeting with one other AID couple. Such networking is offered by some infertility specialists and many RESOLVE chapters.

STRESS

► *After the insemination, my emotions changed back and forth from happy and optimistic to frightened and scared.*

AID is another invasive medical procedure and is also a highly stressful experience. The sperm of another man is inseminated into the wife, and both partners experience many conflicting emotions. Couples may find the insemination treatment a weird event, not the "natural" way of conception they had envisioned.

As a woman begins AID, the worry about both the process itself and about whether pregnancy will occur can sometimes affect her first few menstrual cycles. Stress itself, however, has not been found to be a significant factor in infertility, especially for women. Often couples create even more stress by worrying that their anxiety is preventing pregnancy! If possible try to relieve tension from other more manageable areas of your lives, such as job situations or social obligations.

FANTASIES AND NIGHTMARES

► *I had nightmares about some strange being growing in my abdomen.*

This is a time of intense emotion and transition, so fantasies and nightmares often occur during the AID process. Residual guilt, ambivalence, or anger may surface and sometimes the only safe way to express such emotions is through dreams. As these feelings are resolved, the fantasies and nightmares usually decrease and then stop.

IMPOTENCY AND SEXUAL ISSUES

► *AID brought up feelings of somebody else sleeping with my wife, but I knew how desperately she wanted to carry a child of her own. It was important to her concept of herself as a woman and a mother at that time.*

About half of men who are infertile will experience problems of temporary impotence. It is important to realize that this problem is *quite common* and *only temporary.*

Old infertility feelings can resurface during this time, such as the woman's anger at her husband's inability to impregnate and his guilt, frustration, and feelings of inadequacy due to the medical problem. Feelings of infidelity and jealousy are also common. After all, the woman is being impregnated by another man's sperm. Anger, depression, or jealousy can certainly affect sexuality.

A loss of sexual interest may occur during the first few cycles of AID. A husband may often feel superfluous or unnecessary at this time. His wife goes to the doctor to get the sperm she needs for pregnancy, reinforcing his belief that he is inadequate. The couple may temporarily lose interest in sex and drift apart. In addition myths have been perpetrated about how intercourse should not occur anytime during AID. Although some AID programs advise couples to abstain for certain parts of the cycle, sex is certainly encouraged most of the month.

Love, patience, and understanding are very important during the AID process. This is a time when the couple needs each other the most. Touching, warmth, and togetherness are just as important as intercourse during this stressful time. Having the husband attend and perhaps assist with the inseminations is one way to be close during the process, if that is comfortable for both partners.

Single Women and AID

► *I strongly feel the judgment of others about my decision to try AID. Single women who adopt are considered selfless angels. I think that those of us who attempt pregnancy through AID are viewed as tainted or promiscuous.*

About 10 percent of AID patients are single women, who often encounter disapproval from family and friends, as well as discrimination from the medical profession. Many doctors will not treat unmarried women, or if they do their attitude is cold and judgmental.

A single woman may experience a wide range of reactions during the AID process. On the one hand, she has the freedom to make the decision alone without coping with a male partner's infertility. On the other hand, this freedom can create a sense of isolation and lack of support in the cold, clinical atmosphere of the doctor's office. In addition, some women may not be able to afford monthly inseminations, which may cost between $150 and $200 per try. Since AID is a hit-or-miss process, an infertility problem can go undetected for some time especially if the inseminations are done infrequently.

A number of women's health clinics have created sperm banks for single women desiring AID. Thus, single woman need not seek a physician to act as an intermediary, although many specialists are certainly sympathetic and willing to treat single women. Success rates vary among clinics, so it is wise to research each facility in advance. In addition, some single women are forming groups for emotional support while they go through the AID process.

Issues Unique to the AID Family

► *We have two children, aged 4 and 6, who were conceived by AID. We have already told them that we needed help to get pregnant. When they are ready, we'll tell them about AID and what we know of the donors. We want them to hear it from us and think they should have this knowledge for medical, as well as psychological, reasons. We have been very selective, however, in telling friends and relatives.*

There are probably a quarter of a million to half a million people in the United States today who were conceived by AID. To date there have been no studies done on the long-range effects of AID on the child or the couple.

Some religions do not accept AID as an ethical or legitimate procedure. It is advisable to be quite selective in discussing AID and to be prepared for negative reactions. Many couples feel AID should be kept confidential from extended family and friends but differ on whether to tell their child. They also worry about blood relative challenges to inheritances of AID offspring, particularly in states where laws are vague or unclear.

Some argue that the adoption experience of the last few decades has shown that for most children it is a mistake to conceal their origins. Similarly, they reason, it is wiser to inform a child about AID at the appropriate time. Otherwise the child may later be shocked to discover a different blood type from the parents, perhaps in high school biology class. Others believe it is undesirable and inappropriate to tell their child about AID at any time.

As with adoption, search questions may also arise. Do children have the right to seek their biological fathers? Should the anonymity of a donor be respected in all cases? To further complicate the issue an appellate court in California has recently ruled that, in cases where donor sperm was inseminated by *someone other than a physician,* the donor has paternity rights. Whether this ruling will be upheld in California or be adopted or expanded by other state courts remains to be seen.

Coping Suggestions

► *We found that joking about AID and accepting it as slightly bizarre helped. On the morning of my first treatment, Curt and I woke up, turned to each other, and cracked up. We wondered if the doctor was saving $50 by not using* donor *sperm after all!*

The following suggestions are offered by couples who have been through the AID process:

- Be sure the decision is right for you as a couple—that you are both in agreement and have resolved anger, jealousy, and grief issues before you start AID.

- Throughout the decision-making and treatment process, seek support and counseling from those with firsthand experience of AID.

- Maintain your sense of humor. It is a great tension reliever during AID treatment.

- Make this a special bonding time. Go to the inseminations together if you are comfortable with that. Plan special outings and treats for yourselves during this time.

- There can be ongoing stress after pregnancy and birth, especially if the AID remains secret. This is a lifelong situation that requires continuing patience, love, and understanding.

PART III

Resolutions

CHAPTER 17

Adoption

Not flesh of my flesh
Nor bone of my bone
But still miraculously my own;
Never forget
For a single minute
You didn't grow
Under my heart
But in it.
ANONYMOUS

The practice of adoption, a wonderful and usually joyous resolution to infertility, is as old as humankind. Since prehistoric times, people have adopted children for a variety of reasons. Today adoption gives those who have ached to love and nurture a child the chance to do so. Many fertile families have also chosen to adopt in addition to or instead of bearing biological children. In any case adoption is a highly personal, often intense process that tremendously affects a triad of parties—birthparents, adoptive parents, and adoptees—for a lifetime.

In the past most adoptions in the United States were handled by public or private agencies that had more babies available for adoption than families willing to parent them. Since the 1970s, however, this situation has changed dramatically. Bearing a child outside of marriage, once a social stigma, is gaining wider acceptance, and many single women now intentionally have and keep their babies. More effective and increased use of birth control, as well as liberalized abortion laws, have also significantly reduced the number of unplanned infants who might be placed through adoption.

There are, however, still many children who are older or handicapped in some way and sibling groups available through agency adoption. In addition there are still some birthmothers who wish to place their infants with adoptive families. Some relinquish their babies to agencies for placement, but increasingly, numbers of birthparents are actively participating in the placement of their babies with adoptive couples or individuals. Legal in many, but not all, states, this process is termed *independent* or *private adoption,* and accounts for more than half the adoptions now occurring in the United States.

After interviewing dozens of adoption triad members, it became apparent that each had his or her own feelings and philosophy about the way adoption should be. There are no right answers about adoption. This chapter offers a variety of perspectives and options for the reader's consideration. Further readings and resources are offered in the bibliography and Appendix A.

Making the Decision to Adopt

► *My marriage was only two months old when I had my first surgery. An emergency removal of a badly diseased right ovary and tube was done. I was consumed with the need to get pregnant right away. This has been my year and a half for acting upon, and diligently concentrating on, what is so terribly wrong with me that no child can be realized through my body—being torn apart physically to probe for a cause and mentally trying to adjust to my sorrow and despair.*

Now I see a light growing brighter at the end of this tunnel of infertility. Adoption is my chance to believe again in, and concentrate on, what is good and strong about myself and my marriage. I am out of practice, but am again learning to dwell on what I do have to offer a baby. I am rising above the realization of imperfect physical being, and the suffering this brings, to view myself through adoption as whole again—as the mother of someone who needs me. I am again seeing myself with much to give—if not my uterus to grow in, then my arms to lie in, my love to have, my life to share.

Childlessness is not me. And now I know it does not have to be. I have resolved myself to adoption in mind and heart, and welcome the love it will bring to me. I will be a mother—the realization of a dream.

Most couples who wish to parent assume they will bear one or more biological children. Those who want a large family may imagine adopting a third or fourth child after they experience childbirth. Infertile couples, however, often realize that adoption is the *only* way they can have children and approach this option with a great deal of frustration or grief. Adoption may seem like a last resort to these couples: "If we can't get pregnant, or get too old, then we'll have to adopt."

Making the decision to adopt under these circumstances can be a long, painful process. While deciding whether this is the right solution for you, it is helpful to consider and discuss the difficult issues involved. Both partners might read over the following questions, think about their reactions for a few days, and then compare their feelings.

- Do we feel inadequate, inferior, or incomplete because of our infertility?
- Have we thoroughly grieved for our inability to have a biological child?
- Will we continue to try for a pregnancy after adoption?
- What will we do if we get pregnant while awaiting an adoption?
- Do we feel as excited about adoption as we did about trying for a pregnancy?
- Are we ready, financially and emotionally, to become parents tomorrow, next week, or next month?
- Are we aware that adoption is a lifelong process, a fact that our family must always cope with?
- Are we prepared for the emotional stress of the adoption process?
- Can we afford the costs of private or agency adoption?
- Would we be comfortable in meeting the birthparents and/or maintaining contact with them in the future?
- Do we wish to adopt only an infant? Would we be comfortable with an older child, one with a handicap, or a child of another race?
- What are our reservations? Why haven't we adopted already?
- Are we both sure adoption is the right resolution for us?

Are you in agreement on most of these questions? Or does one partner want to adopt while the other wishes to remain child-free? If you find yourself in accord about adoption, you are ready to begin the process.

► *Don and I had never considered adoption because we had endless hope I could get pregnant. When our treatment ended we felt great relief that the stress and tension were over; yet we were in limbo about our lives. Weren't we five years ago trying to enlarge our family? Had we forgotten our original goal of wanting to give love and security to our child? This haunted us for some time.*

We started talking to adoptive parents, adopted children, and doctors. We phoned friends, read books about adoption, and had long discussions. One evening Don said, "Let's go for it."

From that moment on we worked 110 percent for an adoption, just as we had with our infertility, and there were never any regrets, remorse, or skepticism. We knew it was only a matter of time before we would start our family, our original goal.

Five years is a long labor that a fertile woman will never understand. Three years ago, Don and I were blessed with our adoptive baby daughter, and you can't bring us down from the clouds yet!

On the other hand couples often disagree on a number of issues and feel angry or impatient with each other. Both may already be distressed and exhausted from their infertility experience. At this time it may be difficult to communicate honestly and objectively about adoption.

As they consider adoption, most couples receive a lot of unsolicited advice from friends and relatives. Ignore those who just *know* how "awful, stressful, and impossible" adoption is, or who *guarantee* you'll get pregnant as soon as you adopt. Instead, ask the experts: adoptive parents and the professionals who work in this field. They can give you accurate information, reassurance, and insights about both the stresses and joys of the adoption experience. Many RESOLVE chapters also sponsor preadoption meetings where couples who have adopted share their insights and experience.

Pursuing Both Adoption and Pregnancy

► *We went to an agency group meeting and were told that the wait for an infant would be four years. Having friends who had just gotten a child, we knew it would more likely be five or six years. However, I was only 30, John was 34, and we could still try for a pregnancy. We were just covering all the bases and felt we were taking positive steps forward.*

Some couples may decide to begin the adoption process while continuing their infertility treatment, willing to parent either biologically or through adoption. Others want a larger family and adopt one or more children while trying for a biological child. Whatever your reasons for pursuing both options, it is important to approach adoption with the same careful consideration and soul-searching you gave to pregnancy. To do otherwise is unfair to both yourselves and your adopted child.

Couples who wish to have only one child, or children spaced several years apart, should also weigh this decision carefully. A common myth predicts a pregnancy for every couple who adopts. Actually there is only a small chance (about 5 percent) of such an event, and most likely this spontaneous pregnancy would have happened anyway. But it could happen to you. Are you willing and able to raise two children closely spaced, one child biological and the other adopted? If you are not comfortable with this possibility, you may want to postpone one option while pursuing the other.

Grieving for Your Biological Child

► *I had been unable to admit that I couldn't get pregnant through my own force of will; I could not accept defeat. After this realization, I gradually began to feel more comfortable with the notion of failure. And I could begin to separate failure to get pregnant from failure as a woman or as a person.*

It was at this point that, for the first time, I was able actively to pursue my goal to become a parent. Today my husband and I are the parents of a beautiful, bright, loving 2½-year-old son whom we adopted on the day of his birth.

► *The sadness of not birthing a child still occasionally surfaces. It is, however, not the same wrenching pain as before we adopted Tina. I've made my peace with what happened. The sadness has been put in its place.*

Some infertile couples overcome their desire to have a biological child and stop medical treatment altogether. With enormous relief they end this frustrating quest and channel their energy into adoption. They are again in control of their lives. Their love and devotion deepens and, with time, sexual intimacy is again spontaneous and passionate, associated with love and pleasure rather than pursuing procreation.

Before they can concentrate on adoption, however, most grieve for the loss of the biological child they had hoped to raise. This is often a devastating loss—perhaps compounded by guilt that they waited too long—along with anger at this cruel twist of fate. Accepting adoption as an equally exciting alternative can be a long, difficult process.

OUR FANTASY CHILD For many couples the pregnancy and birth of a child of our flesh is a life's dream. Most of us assume that our biological offspring will be superior specimens with all our best qualities. Few fantasize about a child with a physical handicap or a disagreeable personality. There is also a natural curiosity about our biological child. Would she or he have my nose, your dimples, our artistic bent? Humorously posing an alternative fantasy can put things into perspective.

► *It hit me that there was no reason to assume that this fantasy child was going to get all our good qualities. While playing roulette with these genes, those of our relatives might get the upper hand. I started to laugh right on the freeway. I pictured a little cousin Henry!*

The flip side became apparent. Some pregnant young lady might have all kinds of good things connecting inside her. In our case it was true. We got a cute, wonderful kid. I take the credit whenever he does anything good!

Certainly we would like to pass on our physical traits and emotional chemistries to our children. But when pregnancy is not possible or likely, consider the other qualities you have to offer.

► *What do you really want to pass on to your kids? I feel most grateful to my own parents for emotional, rather than genetic, heritage. I would like to pass on values, love, and feelings to my children, rather than the shape of an ear. I'm not belittling pregnancy. If you can do it, fine. But if you're having problems and shying away from adoption because of the fact that this is not your biological child, it's important to question what you fear.*

Parenting is about having a child. This can be done without a child coming out of you. You don't have to be related to people by blood to love them.

SOCIETY'S BIAS Because our society favors biological parenting over adoption, infertile couples often think that their relatives and friends consider pregnancy the only real way to have a family. As potential grandparents confront their own mortality, they often yearn for biological descendants. They convey this message, subtly or not, to their own children. Couples considering adoption often fear their child would not be treated "like blood" by their extended family. It is important for these couples to seek counsel and perhaps discuss these issues with their extended families.

Usually, of course, once a couple adopts, their relatives and friends fall in love with their special child.

► *Sean is so special, not only to us but to our friends and family who now understand what we went through to have him. He is a special blessing resulting from our infertility. We could not love him more if he were our biological child. He is truly a miracle. He may learn that I didn't carry him, but he knows I am his mother—the one who feeds him, cares for him, and loves him.*

Adoption as a Lifelong Process

► *When I was in my early twenties, I suffered from severe endometriosis, which required surgery to remove my ovaries, tubes and uterus. My husband and I wanted children very much. Fortunately in those days you simply went to an adoption agency and, if you qualified, requested a little girl or boy. We were so lucky to adopt two girls and a boy all in their infancy.*

At first we encountered the usual thoughtless remarks from friends and relatives. But most irritating was the comment, "How lucky those children are that you adopted them!"

Why, from the very first John and I have felt that we are the lucky ones, and we still do! Our children are wonderful people who have given us such joy. Neither of us has ever regretted their adoption or the fact that we did not birth them. They are our children in every way that matters.

When they were each about 3 years old, we matter-of-factly told each of them that we were unable to have children and that we adopted them. After that, we rarely discussed it. We didn't consider them "special" because they were adopted. From the very beginning, we thought of and treated them as our own children.

As my children grew up, each experienced different emotions about adoption. I remember my little boy, at just 5 or 6 years old, being very angry with his biological mother for giving him up. When I explained that she just couldn't afford to raise him, he muttered, "Well, she could have got a job!"

We have been the happiest of families. I never thought much about adopting my children until my oldest daughter got pregnant. When she first told me the wonderful news, we looked at each other and cried. I realized that the birth experience was one thing we couldn't discuss and compare notes on. This daughter is also quite adamant about not ever seeing her biological parents. She requested that the adoption agency put a letter in her file that states her desire not to be contacted by either party. She told me of this decision one Mother's Day when she explained that I am the only mother she has.

My youngest daughter is curious about her birthparents. She has told me, "Mom, I don't really want to meet them, or have them in my life. I would just like to see what they look like." I told her that I am secure in her love and understand her curiosity. I will help her locate these people if this is what she wants.

I have never felt less of a woman because I did not bear a child. My husband and I have had a very happy, wonderful marriage of 34 years. For those who are infertile and wish to have children, I strongly recommend adoption. For us, it has been a very happy, wonderful experience.

Adopting a child, while a resolution to infertility, is more importantly the first step of a lifelong experience. Like biological parenting, adoption brings the laughter, tears, and exhaustion of raising a family. It also carries unique joys, stresses, and losses. Viewing adoption in a realistic light beforehand can prevent a lot of misunderstanding and grief after the fact.

The adoption triad consists of the birthparents, adoptive parents, and the adopted child. All three parties retain feelings about this adoption for the rest of their lives. There is, however, no right or normal reaction to adoption.

For the infertile couple, adoption is usually viewed as a resolution to a heartbreaking problem. In a sense their infertility will be solved by adoption; no longer will they be childless. They are, however, parenting the birthchild of others, not one of their bodies. Those who do not have biological children may grieve for that loss and carry residual feelings about their infertility throughout their lives.

► *I don't think it is easy for a woman to accept the fact that a life may never grow within her. But it is harder to imagine never experiencing the joy and pleasure of raising a child. I will always wish that I had actually carried Sean and given birth to him. I feel the loss of those nine months even while I cherish the blessing of having him as my son for the rest of my life. But I have come to realize that pregnancy lasts a very short time; raising a child lasts a lifetime.*

Adoptive parents may also fear future contact from the birthparents or that their child may someday want to meet them. If a reunion does occur, some adoptive parents worry that their child may become closely acquainted with or even prefer the birthparents. Many fear any link with a biological parent will result in a loss of their child's love.

The birthparents (and perhaps their families) are struggling with the loss of a child and part of their genetic line. In many cases the birthmother is a young, single girl, and her baby is both families' first grandchild. Some birthfathers run away from the problem; others, along with their families, share feelings of love for the child and take an active role in the adoption process.

Often birthmothers are without financial resources and education; some have been rejected or abandoned by the child's father. One therapist described many of the birthmothers she counsels as "floundering, frightened, and overwhelmed by their circumstances." Throughout their pregnancies many of these women are ambivalent about their decision to relinquish their babies. Indeed birthing a child is such a monumental event that it is hard to predict how any woman will feel until she delivers her baby. Many of these women, however, have great feelings of love toward their unborn child and have continued their pregnancies because of it. Because they are unable to parent at this time, relinquishing the child is usually a painful, wrenching decision that can leave a lifetime of ambivalent feelings. Some later suffer the added pain of not bearing other children.

► *Like me, I think most birthmothers never get over relinquishing their child. After carrying your baby and feeling that life bounding within you, you can't just forget about your child or stop wondering how he is doing throughout his life. This is particularly painful if this choice is made from family pressure or economic necessity.*

As their lives progress, many birthparents come to terms with their relinquishment decision, although feelings resurface over the years. Some yearn to meet their biological child when he or she is an adult. Although most fear rejection from the adoptive parents and their birthchild, some attempt to locate the child anyway.

Most adoptees eventually learn they were relinquished by their biological parents. Although individual reactions vary, depending on the age and temperament of the child, the fact of being adopted can evoke confusing and frightening feelings of abandonment and loss of identity. Some adoptees who haven't seen pictures of their birthmothers describe an eerie feeling that they weren't really born. Identity issues often resurface during adolescence and can be compounded when the child does not physically resemble his adoptive family.

► *My adolescence was quite painful. Along with the normal identity issues all teenagers experience, I also wondered why I carried one family's name and another's heredity; why my biological parents didn't want me; whether I looked like them.*

Such questions may eventually lead an adoptee to search for his or her birthparents (and genetic heredity) and perhaps arrange a reunion. This meeting can raise many feelings: hope of discovery and reconciliation, fear of another rejection by the birthparents, and pain that this gesture is hurting the adoptive family. The need to search, however, should not be equated with a loss of love for the adoptive parents. Instead the child is looking for a tie to physical origins, which may or may not result in an emotional bond.

Some triad members give little thought to their adoption experience, while others report continuing feelings of anger, love, abandonment, gratitude, and sadness. These are not emotions that should or can be fixed. For these people adoption is a lifelong challenge. The Post Adoption Center for Education and Research (PACER), founded by Dirck Brown (an adoptee) is devoted to supporting *all* triad members. They offer many services, including literature, support groups, conferences, and referrals (see Appendix A).

Public and Private Agency Adoption

► *My first call was to an adoption agency that told me my husband was just at their cutoff age for applications and that if we applied that day it would probably take at least 5 years to adopt a healthy infant. The waiting lists were that long. I hung up totally discouraged.*

► *Just a few months after we filed our application we were surprised by a call from the county adoption service. They had a baby girl who needed a home. Were we still interested? Were we!! We madly scrambled for clothes, crib, and diapers and brought her home a few days before Christmas.*

Adoption agencies are licensed, state-regulated private or public organizations that coordinate the adoption process between birthparents who wish to relinquish their child (or those whose children are removed from their homes by the state) and couples or individuals seeking to adopt a child. The process begins with the birthparents' relinquishment of legal custody of their child to the agency. After carefully screening prospective parents the agency places the child with an adoptive couple or individual. The final stage of agency adoption occurs with the transfer of legal custody by the court to the adoptive parents.

Agency adoptions are considered safer than independent ones because, in most cases, the birthparents have surrendered their legal rights upon relinquishing the child to the agency. Unless they can prove the relinquishment papers were signed under fraudulent conditions or duress, it is highly unlikely that the court would return the child to them after placement. In a very small percentage of adoptions the child may be returned to the birthparents after the consent is signed but before the court finalizes the adoption.

In cases where one or both birthparents have not signed relinquishment papers, the agency will initiate legal proceedings to terminate parental rights. In most instances the child is not placed with an adoptive family until he or she is legally free. In some agency placements, however, the child has not been legally freed by both birthparents. For example, the agency may have been unable to locate the birthfather and obtain his signature for relinquishment. The child is then placed in a fost-adopt arrangement until the legal procedures are completed. In this situation there is a small chance that there will be a court hearing for custody. Before placement the agency will notify the adoptive parents of the situation and the possible risk of losing the child.

Fees

Adoption agencies charge a fee for their services that varies depending on whether the organization is public (e.g., county) or private (e.g., church-related). All reputable agencies conduct informational meetings to discuss their operating procedures and fees. Sliding scale fees are usually offered and some employers and insurance companies cover all or part of the adoption expense.

Ask your specialist, state or county department of social services, or RESOLVE chapter for referrals to reputable agencies.

Qualifying as an Adoptive Parent

► *The agencies willing to work with us had a waiting list of several years. We would also have to expose ourselves body and soul in order to qualify. Before considering us, they wanted a reason for my infertility. I was unwilling to discuss it; after three years of tests, I had no medical reason. I was just "different" and I was angry. This stage of anger has been the most difficult for me to face and resolve. I'm sure it has impacted our subsequent attempts at adoption.*

► *We had heard that it was difficult to adopt through an agency and that the social workers were veterans of the system who really put you through the wringer. We had, however, made up our minds to go through whatever was necessary; we really wanted to be parents. From the beginning, though, the county staff made us feel comfortable. They wanted to know about our family backgrounds and occupations. Our initial meeting lasted more than two hours but the time flew by. We passed through the first screening and two more appointments were made: one with only my husband, the other in our home.*

Before you can adopt a child through an agency, you must meet their requirements as suitable parents. The criteria for qualifying varies with each agency. In fact there are so few babies available that many individuals and couples are either not accepted or placed on long waiting lists. Such a rejection should not be taken personally; there just aren't enough babies available through agency adoption to meet the demand.

The qualifying process can be difficult. You may not be accustomed to the scrutiny and investigation required, and anger about your infertility may resurface. After all there are no qualifying tests required for pregnancy.

Most agencies call this qualifying or screening procedure the "home study process," which begins with a detailed questionnaire regarding your income level, age, medical history, living environment, and reasons for wishing to adopt. The process also requires one or more informational meetings, several interviews at the agency, and a home visit. A social worker will work with you during your home study.

Most couples fear that the social worker has a great deal of power and may make subjective judgments about their ability to parent and provide a good home. Understandably they want to make a good impression and pass the test. The infertile couple is also being evaluated at a time when they feel quite vulnerable. This is a tense situation where misunderstandings can occur.

► *Sessions with our worker were emotional and not always positive or productive as I tried to deal with my anger. I was trying to accept my own incapabilities but angrily refused to let go of the hope that I might solve my infertility without help from an agency. I resented the power our worker had over us, the fact that I was not in control, the questions we had to answer, and the degree to which we had to expose ourselves. After all most people didn't have to go through all this; they just got pregnant. We had to deal with our own feelings and doubts while being judged suitable or unsuitable to be parents.*

Each social worker is an individual and every agency has its criteria for "good parents." Most agree, however, that emotional maturity, stability, a loving home, and a strong desire to parent are most important. The social worker will observe how the couple has accepted their infertility and whether they feel inadequate because of it.

► *Our worker, Jenny, talked with us at length about our infertility. We were very honest and told her of the surgeries and futile months of trying to conceive. She also asked about my background, upbringing, and family history. We felt good about her: here was a person sincere in her questions who would help us find a child.*

The social worker will also note whether a couple is entering the adoption process while still in grief and will question their intentions if they get pregnant while awaiting adoption or shortly thereafter. Many couples panic when they suspect a fertility problem and rush into the adoption process without careful thought.

The agency is also interested in the couple's marital relationship. Are they open and flexible to the changes parenting will bring? How do they settle differences? Most workers also want to ensure that couples are well informed about adoption and aware that it is different from biological parenthood. They will ask how the couple would cope, over the years, with the child's curiosity about adoption and birthparents.

In most cases prospective adoptive parents and their social workers like and respect each other. It sometimes happens, however, that the entire interview process is unpleasant and upsetting. You may have a personality conflict with your worker, feel overly investigated, or receive an unfavorable evaluation. In this event you might discuss your feelings with other agency personnel and perhaps request that another social worker be assigned to your case.

THE HOME VISIT

► *The days before the home visit were filled with anxiety, happiness, and a great sense of relief. We had finally done something positive for ourselves for a change. We cleaned, cleaned, cleaned! Our case worker was a warm, wonderful woman, and soon we were all laughing and talking. She asked to see our home. I showed her all around, including the room we were saving for our child. It had not been painted, wallpapered, or cleaned since we moved in a year before. We couldn't bear to fix it up until we really had a child. We adopted a little boy soon after and remain grateful for our worker's kindness and help.*

The screening process usually involves a series of interviews with at least one "home visit." The social worker is interested in the living environment, as well as how the prospective parents interact at home. Most couples are, naturally, nervous before this visit and worry that their home is inadequate. Once the interview has begun, however, most find that the visit goes smoothly.

Placement

► *We called the final set of papers the "soul-searching" set. The questions asked what kind of child would we accept into our home; which handicaps and medical conditions we could handle; what racial backgrounds were acceptable. We had to dig deep into ourselves and ask for the first time, what kind of child could we see ourselves parent.*

After completing the interview process acceptable couples or individuals are placed in a waiting pool until a child is available. At this point you must both decide which race and age and which physical, mental, and emotional handicaps are acceptable. Most agencies predict a long wait (four to eight years) for a Caucasian infant and *almost immediate placement for a sibling group or an older or handicapped child* (especially with public agencies). Most agencies prefer to place children with families of the same ethnic heritage. Today many nonwhite families can be ethnically matched with children within a few months.

Length of wait may also depend on the preferences of the birthmother. Increasingly agencies are incorporating her input into the selection process. A birthmother may indicate a preference for religious affiliation or presence of a sibling in the adoptive home. Many agencies feel this participation reassures the birthmother that she is making the right choice and helps her live with the decision. On request some agencies also arrange a meeting of the parties before the birth. Although each case is evaluated individually, more openness about triad members' identity is occurring in agency as well as independent adoption.

Once placement occurs, there is usually a supervision period of 6 to 12 months. To ensure that each family member is adjusting well to the adoption, the agency will contact and visit your home during this interim. If the placement is acceptable to agency, parents, and child, the adoption will be legally finalized in court. If not, agency personnel will work with the family to resolve the problem.

Biological Father's Legal Rights

Recent court decisions and statutes, such as the Uniform Paternity Act of 1975, are changing the legal rights of biological fathers in the adoption process. Both public and private adoption agencies now make a determined effort to have both biological parents sign relinquishment papers before the child is placed. The biological father may also be given the option of denying paternity or waiving further notice to him of adoption planning. If he cannot be located, the agency tries to trace him through the Department of Motor Vehicles, his last three known addresses, and his social security number. The adoptive parents are notified whether the birthfather has been located and if he has consented to relinquishment.

Interracial Adoptions

► *We adopted a little girl while living in India and two children of mixed black and Caucasian parentage after we returned to the U.S. Our children are now 15, 19, and 22.*

Our families were strongly opposed to our decisions at first and the early days were quite painful. It has taken many years for them to come around.

We've lived in several different cities over the years and found racism and cruelty in each place as well as love and acceptance. When our children were small, strangers would approach us and ask if these were my kids. When I nodded, they would stare and ask, "What did you do that for?" I was furious that they were so cruel in front of my kids and wanted to protect my children. We've also had criticism from both white and black acquaintances.

The early teenage years were pretty tough at times, with both racial and identity issues to confront at once! My kids were also confused about which racial group to identify with both in and out of school. I think anyone considering interracial adoption should give careful thought to their decision. The fact of adoption is a constant visible issue in an interracial family.

We love our kids and wouldn't trade them. I feel we've weathered the tough times and will remain a close family in the years to come.

Although many social workers recommend that children be placed with racially compatible families, interracial adoption still does occur. A couple considering this option must be quite honest with themselves. That they are an adopted family is highly visible to the rest of the world; they cannot "pass" as other ethnically matched adopted families. In these families parents and children with different racial characteristics must bond with each other. This internal pressure is magnified by our society's racism, creating a lifetime of tensions unique to the interracial family. Several good books about this subject and support organizations for families choosing this type of adoption are listed in the bibliography and Appendix A.

Fost-Adopt Programs

► *Only six weeks after our home study, we received a call about a 2-month-old infant, Gary. We were interviewed by four social workers and were scared to death. We tried to psych them out. What questions would they ask? The only one I remember is "How soon can you be ready?" They passed us pictures of the baby and I passed them right back. I couldn't bear to look at them for long. He was so beautiful—big eyes, olive complexion, and dark hair. He could have been our biological son.*

They explained Gary's history. His mother had abandoned him at birth, but he was not legally free yet. He would be in the fost-adopt program until the court took the parents' legal rights away. We were one of 250 couples screened for Gary. Several others were interviewed, but we were chosen! Shock, tears, and relief overwhelmed us. We took him home two months later.

Gary was 16 months old before he was legally freed by the court. It was a very difficult time. Then it took another eight months before his adoption was finalized by the court.

Since that time, we've had another son placed with us through fost-adopt. Tommy had similar circumstances at birth as Gary, but his birthmother did relinquish rights to him. We did not have to go through the hearing process and are now in the six-month waiting period for finalization of his adoption.

The most important message we have for others is that there are children available through county fost-adopt programs. We felt embraced by the system, were treated with respect, and thought all legal matters were attended to properly. We never felt alone or confused.

Fost-adopt programs are usually administered by county social service agencies. A child who has been surrendered by or removed from the biological parents can be placed in a home as a foster child. There may be a delay, while the county completes its investigation and prepares reports and recommendations, before legal proceedings begin and the adoption is finalized in court. In cases where the child is not yet legally freed for adoption, there is a small risk (usually less than 10 percent) that he or she will be returned to the birthparents. Check with your state or county department of social services for further information about fost-adopt programs.

Special Needs Adoption

Special needs adoptions include older children (usually over 6 years of age), those of all ages with handicaps of a physical, emotional, or psychological nature, and sibling groups. There is usually a short wait and low initial expense for this type of adoption. However, greater emotional energy and higher financial cost may be required to raise special needs children.

Older children can be especially challenging. Many have been abandoned, rejected, and perhaps physically or sexually abused several times in their young lives. When placing these children, most agencies look for parents who understand their history and the behavior it may elicit. Experienced parents are usually better able to cope with such demands; a special needs adoption may be an overwhelming place to begin parenting.

AASK America (Aid to Adoption of Special Kids) is a California-based organization that facilitates special needs adoptions and offers counseling and referral services to interested families (see Appendix A). They also offer a program that matches adoptive parents over the age of 21 with a compatible special needs child.

International Adoption

► *After my unsuccessful surgery Steve surprised me by suggesting adoption. We decided to adopt a Korean child and have asked for a girl. With finally terminating our treatment, and our orientation meeting with the agency coming up, I feel we are at the same point for the first time in three years. I already love the tiny child I will adopt and it seems very unimportant that she be born from our bodies. After much pain and struggle I now feel my infertility has made me a unique and special person. Resolving with foreign adoption has reinforced those feelings.*

International adoption, in which a U.S. couple or individual adopts a child from another country, is becoming more popular. Because of long agency waits and increasing competition for independent adoptions, many U.S. couples are drawn to the idea of parenting a child from another culture. Some couples also feel that their infertility struggle has given them sensitivity and compassion toward others and created this special opportunity for having a child.

These adoptions are often handled through private agencies and involve the U.S. Department of Immigration. A home study is required and a couple's motivation to adopt a foreign child will be carefully evaluated before they are accepted by an agency. As with any type of adoption, you must be cautious about selecting an agency. Your county social services department or RESOLVE chapter can provide referrals; a partial list of international adoption agencies is also included in Appendix A.

Some U.S. families have taken the initiative themselves of finding a child from another country to adopt (private intercountry adoption). They arrange for a home study, negotiate with an agency or orphanage abroad, meet that country's legal requirements and other red tape, and then pick up their child in his or her native country. You can obtain more information about this type of international adoption from the Organization for a United Response (OURS), listed in Appendix A.

Either kind of international adoption can be quite costly. Airfare from the home country, along with immigration, escort, and agency fees must be paid by the adopting parents.

Before embarking on this process, be advised that there are several myths surrounding international adoption: that the children are all orphans and do not have any relatives remaining in their native land, that they have not been abused or neglected, and that the child will easily assimilate into our culture.

In many cases the child was relinquished to an agency by one or both birthparents, who, along with their extended family, are very much alive. As such children grow up, they will probably be curious about their ancestry, origins, and native culture. You could face the same search issues as other adoptive families. In the meantime you must consider providing information about the history and culture of the child's native country and incorporate this heritage into your family life.

Many of these children have also suffered from hunger, disease, and physical or sexual abuse. Upon entering a new and strange society, culture shock is also common. In many ways, these are special needs children and present similar challenges to adoptive parents.

As with interracial adoption, your family may confront intolerance and racism from relatives, friends, and community. Are both you and your mate able to cope with such bigotry and cruelty?

Sealed Records

In most states, agency adoption records are sealed when the adoption is legally finalized in court. This preserves the anonymity of the triad members. Some of these parties prefer the permanent secrecy of closed records. Others, frustrated in their attempts to find birthparents or adoptees, favor legislative changes to open these records to concerned parties.

Agencies that have handled thousands of adoptions over the years report an overwhelming number of requests for identifying information from all triad members. These agencies are bound by the laws of confidentiality and cannot disclose the identities of any party or even any nonidentifying information (such as medical histories, ethnic heritage, age of birthparents at the adoptee's birth, etc.) without the written permission of *all* triad members. An increasing number of states, however, will open sealed records when the adoptee reaches majority. Check with an adoption attorney or your state's department of social services for further assistance.

Independent Adoption: A Northern California Case Study

► *I pursued an independent adoption lead while lying in my hospital bed recovering from a surgery that left me, like my husband, clinically sterile. The lead did not work out, but it did convince me that adoption was our answer and that there was a child out there for us. Nothing was going to stop me from finding him or her.*

We told all our friends and family about our decision and joined an adoption support group. We were able to verbalize, not only to the group but also to each other, all our fears and apprehensions about adoption and finally conclude that it was not birthing, but parenting that we wanted more than anything else. As couple after couple began to search privately for infants to adopt, we gained more courage to reach out and test our vulnerability again. This time we were operating with a strong support system and that made all the difference.

Although independent adoption has been practiced for decades, in past years most U.S. adoptions were handled by agencies. In the 1960s, up to 13,000 adoptions occurred each year. More babies were available than parents willing to adopt them and nearly three-quarters of these adoptions were handled by agencies. Today a greater demand exists for adoptable babies than ever before. The baby boom generation, many of whom deferred childbearing in their twenties, are reaching their late childbearing years. Those who can't get pregnant face a dwindling supply of babies to adopt. The majority of couples who wish to adopt now use independent adoption to enlarge their families. Between 1975 and 1985 nearly 30,000 independent adoptions occurred.

In the independent adoption process, the birthparents and adoptive parents arrange the adoption themselves, usually with the assistance of an intermediary such as an attorney. An adoption agency is not involved in the selection of the adoptive parents, although the state's department of social services does perform a home study to validate the birthparent's choice.

The child is placed directly with the adoptive parents, often immediately after discharge from the hospital or shortly thereafter. In most cases the adoptive parents' attorney performs the necessary legal steps. Some birthmothers, if they are financially able, retain their own attorney to represent their interests.

Sometimes the parties mutually decide to meet one or more times. Some birthmothers stay with the adopting couple during part of their pregnancies, and some adoptive parents attend the birth of the child. On the other hand some birthparents or adoptive parents choose *not* to meet face to face. In any case the names and addresses of each party are known to the other. This openness is a radical departure from the secrecy that has shrouded adoption for the last few decades, and it raises many questions.

Several northern California families have generously shared their perspectives and experiences for this text. If you are considering independent adoption, be sure to obtain current, accurate legal information about your state's laws, and those of the birthparents if they reside elsewhere.

How to Adopt a Child Independently

► *Nobody wants to find a baby for you as much as you do, and there are birthparents who want to find good homes for their babies. Tell everyone you can think of that you want to adopt a baby.*

You have something to offer too. You may think, "I'm so needy. I want to solve my problem." You will be solving your problem, true, but you'll also be solving someone else's. You're providing a good home. You're going to all this trouble to have a child because you think you can be a damn good parent. That's something to offer a pregnant woman.

Write letters to doctors and those who counsel pregnant women. If you send enough letters to enough people, you will find the right one.

In many states birthparents have a legal right to place their own child for adoption. Some couples find a child to adopt by themselves. Others pay a fee to an independent adoption program to help them with the process. Either way many people have happily adopted infants at birth, or shortly afterward, through independent adoption.

Most people, however, feel overwhelmed by the task and wonder how to contact pregnant women interested in private adoption. Once they have a lead, they worry about making a good impression on the birthmother. Many infertile couples already feel inadequate and fear rejection and further disappointment with private adoption. It is important to realize that, just as most couples don't get pregnant on the first or second try, it may take adoptive parents several leads to find the right child. Those who enter the process with flexibility and determination to find the right arrangement usually succeed.

Fortunately there are many resources for both information and support. Thousands of successful independent adoptions have occurred. The experts in this field—adoptive parents, attorneys, and birthparents—offer the following advice to interested couples.

STEP 1: TELL EVERYONE YOU KNOW THAT YOU WANT TO ADOPT A CHILD Some couples fear "going public" about their infertility and dread the reactions of friends and family. This step, however, often yields a twofold benefit:

1. It can lead directly to a child. For example, your aunt may work with a man whose friend's niece wants to find a home for her unborn child. Many such leads come from friends of friends.

2. It is often a relief to acknowledge your fertility problem publicly. Friends and relatives, whether or not they were aware of your infertility, now have a positive way to help. Most will react favorably to your decision and lend assistance and moral support.

STEP 2: ENGAGE A REPUTABLE ATTORNEY Find an attorney in your state experienced with both the legal aspects and the emotional issues of independent adoption. These attorneys usually do not find babies for couples but provide expert legal advice about adoption laws and perform the required paperwork once the couple has reached an agreement with a birthmother.

Legal fees for independent adoptions vary depending on the complexity. For example, there may be negotiations with several different birthmothers before one lead works out. Most attorneys charge an hourly rate.

STEP 3: COMPOSE A LETTER

► *Independent adoption meant composing a personal letter and mailing it to people I did not know: doctors, lawyers, hospitals and women's centers. Could I handle this amount of exposure? Did I have enough energy left to compose and mail a thousand letters? Could I handle the returned mail and contacts from people upset with my method? How would I handle contact from a birthmother? How would I cope if this didn't work? All of these thoughts scared me, but I wanted control and I found release for my anger in working in this direction.*

With the assistance of an attorney I composed our letter; with the help of my husband I mailed a thousand of them. I also realized I now had to direct my energy elsewhere while waiting for a positive reply.

Most couples compose a one-page letter to mail nationwide to those in contact with birthmothers wishing to place a child. These include family practitioners, social workers, obstetricians, clergy, high school counselors, abortion counselors, and college student health services. Some couples purchase preprinted mailing labels of these professionals from independent adoption services; others consult telephone directories. Professional directories may also be helpful but sometimes contain outdated information.

There is no perfect or magic letter. Every couple is special, and your letter should reflect your uniqueness. Most people include a natural and relaxed picture. Instead of looking rich or beautiful it is more important to look warm, happy, and in love with each other.

The text should include information about yourselves, such as occupation, age, address, and so forth. You might also include a short sentence or two about your fertility problem and whether it is likely that you will bear a child. Most important, however, is to let your personalities, creativity, and sincerity show. Express your feelings about having children and emphasize those qualities that would make you good parents. Remember that in most cases you are trying to reach a young woman and/or her doctor or lawyer. What will demonstrate to them that you are stable, secure, and loving potential parents?

Include phone numbers for both your attorney and your own home. Indicate any preferences for contact. Some birthmothers will want to speak with you directly; others will want to talk only with your attorney.

The following sample letter provides an example of one format to use. Personalize your letter to convey your own uniqueness and desire to parent.

► *We are John and Susan Jones. We love kids but are unable to have our own. We have pursued all the medical treatments available without any success. After a lot of tears and soul-searching, we have realized that we can forgo pregnancy. It is parenting that we want to experience in our lives.*

We live in a small, pleasant rural community in northern California. John is an engineer and Susan is a graphic artist. We have a comfortable home and an income sufficient for a family of three. We are in our midthirties and love art, hiking, good books, and river rafting.

If you know of a young woman who would like to find an adoptive home for her child, please contact our attorney, Sam Johnson, 111 Main St., San Francisco, CA (415) 555-5555 or call us at home (916) 555-5555. Thank you.

STEP 4: FIND THE RIGHT LEAD After mailing your letters, you should receive some leads by phone or mail. Some may not work out. Eventually, however, most determined couples locate the right birthmother and, usually through an attorney, reach mutual agreement about adopting her child and payment for reasonable expenses. At this point the parties may decide to meet. Some adoptive parents even invite the birthmother to visit their home and perhaps stay for a few days or longer; some attend the birth. In other cases either or both both parties may not want a meeting.

After reaching agreement you all wait for the birth. It is common for everyone to feel apprehensive and worry that the other party will change their mind. In most cases this does not happen. The adoptive couple is usually notified shortly before the birth or immediately thereafter.

STEP 5: PAY LEGITIMATE COSTS OF INDEPENDENT ADOPTION The adopting couple may legally pay for reasonable living, medical, and counseling expenses for the birthmother and child. Total adoption costs will vary in each case and are itemized down to the last cent to the court. Your attorney may disburse these payments, or you can pay the birthmother directly. Most of these costs will be known in advance, although medical expenses may increase if complications occur or a cesarean birth is necessary. An accountant can advise you on which, if any, adoption expenses are tax-deductible.

Adoptive parents do not have to agree to any proposal or expense with which they are uncomfortable. It is important, however, to understand that if a birthmother changes her mind, *you do not have a contractual right to sue her for any expenses already paid.*

It is also important to differentiate between a legal, independent adoption and an illegal, or "black market," adoption, which involves sums (sometimes $10,000 or more per item) for unexplained costs. The intermediary, usually an attorney, is legally entitled only to reasonable fees for services and the birthmother only to reasonable living expenses and health care and counseling fees. If you are in doubt, seek advice from your state's department of social services or another reputable adoption attorney.

STEP 6: UNDERTAKE THE LEGAL PROCESS In California a woman who wishes to relinquish her child signs an "infant dismissal report" after the baby's birth. This form is prepared by the hospital and releases the baby directly to the adopting parents. Although this paper protects the hospital, it does not give the adoptive parents legal rights to the child. After they take the baby home, their attorney files a "petition for adoption" with the court.

The department of social services then has 45 working days to interview all parties to the adoption. During their interview, most birthparents sign the "consent to adoption" forms in the presence of an agent of the California State Department of Social Services, or, if out of state, before a notary public. A birthmother residing out of state is sometimes interviewed by the appropriate state agency in her area, or by telephone or letter.

At any time until the consent to adoption has been signed the birthparents have the right to change their minds and the baby will automatically be returned to them. In private adoption many adoptive parents have the baby with them from birth; they run the small risk (about 5 percent) that the child will be reclaimed by one or both birthparents. Each state's laws vary regarding the rights of the biological father in the private adoption process and custody of the child if he is opposed to the adoption.

Once the consent to adoption has been signed, it may not be withdrawn without a court hearing based solely on the best interests of the child. Although such hearings rarely occur, adoptive parents have as good a chance as the birthparents to retain custody of the child.

During the interview process there is also an investigation by the department of social services, which includes a home visit by a social worker. The goal of this visit is to verify the birthmother's placement choice. Only in extreme cases would the social worker recommend against placement.

STEP 7: RECEIVE THE FINAL ADOPTION DECREE Depending on the court's calendar, the adoption is legally finalized about six months from the time the original petition is filed. The adoptive parents and their attorney appear before a judge and a final adoption decree is granted. This decree is exactly the same in independent and agency-handled adoptions.

Independent Adoption Services

In the last few years many private organizations have been created to facilitate independent adoptions. They offer a range of services including the sale of mailing lists of possible contacts, legal assistance, and counseling for both parties. Many couples and individuals have adopted children with the help of such services and enthusiastically recommend them. Others, however, have had negative experience with such organizations and spent precious time and dollars without finding a single lead.

Be very careful in selecting such a service. You must ensure that the organization is reputable and ethical in its procedures. Check with your state's department of social services or RESOLVE for recommendations.

When Independent Adoption Falls Through

► *After five and a half years of marriage, we finally adopted our daughter who is now 11 years old. But before her, we brought home a baby boy through private adoption. We lost him after ten days; his birthmother wanted him back. I felt so punished, like we had done something wrong.*

When our daughter was 2½, we found out about yet another baby. This, too, was a private adoption. We had her seven weeks until we lost her the Monday before Thanksgiving. I still hurt over losing her. I felt as if doomsday had set in. Her room remained the same for four months. I felt so alone and abandoned. I kept getting a gnawing sensation in my upper stomach and it remained there for five years.

Although it is a rare occurrence (less than 5 percent of independent adoptions), a birthparent sometimes demands and wins the return of the child before the the adoption is legally finalized. Although most couples successfully adopt another child afterward, this is nonetheless an event of enormous trauma to both the couple and the child. Bonding occurs immediately and the loss of a child from the family after 1 day or 100 is a tragic event.

Those who have endured the stresses of infertility and the adoption process are especially vulnerable to yet another crisis. Although the baby did not die, there has been a loss. The dreams, hopes, and love showered on that baby by the adoptive parents do die. It is natural that a deep and painful grief follows.

Having a lead fall through can also be devastating. Even though infertility has taught them not to hope too much, a couple finds a birthmother who is sure she wants to place her baby for adoption. They hope and then slowly dream the baby will be theirs. A lead can fall through an hour later or a few days after the birth. In the following story, one woman shares such an experience:

► *Early last week our caseworker called us: "We think we might have a baby for you." The baby's background matched ours. As a racially mixed couple we were astonished and delighted! It was due any day. The mother felt sure that adoption was the right choice for her, and she hadn't seen the father for months. It seemed a dream we had hardly dared to dream was coming true. One moment we tried to suppress joy and excitement; the next, fear and anticipated depression.*

Three days ago we learned the baby was a healthy boy (we already have a girl!) and that his mother had left the hospital without him. Both our hope and fear were stronger. This morning she changed her mind and decided to keep him.

Inside I am raging with loss; at the same time I feel numb and dulled. We had made secret arrangements. I borrowed a bassinet, saying it was for a friend. We had told only two friends so that we could have someone to talk to, and now I can't bring myself to call them to say we didn't get the baby. We made social plans for the next few weeks, privately telling each other with suppressed delight that we might have to cancel them! Now I feel miserable that we can keep those dates, that I'll have time to put in a winter garden after all.

One part of my brain has been paralyzed these last days, while the rest of me mechanically cooks, cleans, goes to meetings, and writes reports. Was I more afraid of the telephone ringing or of it not ringing?

Our little girl, adopted almost two years ago, was a miracle that did happen. We had hardly dared hope for her, and she came true. Every day we marvel at her: Isn't she wonderful? Isn't she incredible? Isn't she the dearest child ever?

These are the parts of the lecture to myself:

If things worked out the way we had hoped, we might have brought home a baby tonight(!), a brother for our daughter, a son for us. Instead we will spend the evening together with our precious daughter. In our lives of immense good fortune, this is really a small, fleeting sadness.

Before we had our daughter, we went through four "almosts." Now that we have her, we can't help but feel that she is the right child for us, and that we are the right parents for her. It seems so natural and perfectly fitting that she should be in our family. If we had gotten one of those other children, we wouldn't have her!

We must hope that this proves to be the right decision for this baby boy and his mother. It's tempting to feel that we would have been better parents. We must let go of this self-righteousness and wish them, from our hearts, a bright future.

It is true that in an independent adoption, you may lose the child. No one, however, gets a child without some risk. Pregnancy itself is a risky business, with a 20 percent chance of a miscarriage or other type of loss. "Anyone who is brave enough to get pregnant," one adoptive father maintains, "is brave enough to take the risk of independent adoption."

The Adoptive Family

Once an adoption is legally finalized, a new family is created. Because their family was formed through adoption, they face several lifelong issues.

A Continuing Family Dialogue

Most experts recommend that parents tell their child, in an honest and straightforward manner appropriate to her or his age, about the adoption. It is not only difficult but also inadvisable to keep this fact a secret from a child, who may painfully discover the truth from someone else.

Many families begin this dialogue when their child is about 3, using one of the excellent children's adoption books. They explain that children come into families by birth or adoption. Neither is better than the other; they're both special. Your child has come into this family through love: yours and his or her birthmother's.

► *Since Anne was about 3 years old, we have talked about her adoption and occasionally read together the letter her birthmother wrote to her about why she gave Anne to us. It is absolutely beautiful, very sad, and leaves no question about her love for Anne.*

One day, when Anne was about 5, I was driving her and a friend, Jenny, to a party. I heard Jenny say to Anne, "I came out of my mommy's tummy and you didn't!"

Anne was very quiet. I asked Jenny if she knew what adoption meant.

She answered, "Yeah, Anne's real mommy didn't have time to take care of her so she gave her away."

Later I spoke with Anne about her friend's remarks. I asked her if she'd like me to read her birthmother's letter to Jenny. She liked this idea.

A few days later, I read the letter to Jenny. She was pleased we shared this with her and said she now understood more about adoption. The next day Anne told her teacher that she is a lucky girl: She has two mommies who love her.

If our family had not openly talked about Anne's adoption over the years, I'm afraid she would have been very hurt by Jenny's remarks. We might not have thought of this solution and would have missed another rich experience with each other.

As a parent you are the best judge of how often to discuss adoption with your child. He or she may ask you questions about the birthparents from time to time. Many parents find the counsel of adoptive parents of older children, their pediatrician, or a trusted psychologist or therapist helpful in dealing with this curiosity. A dialogue about both parents' and child's fears and hopes can result in honest and sensitive communication and pave the way for a healthy relationship throughout their lives.

Open Adoption

► *When we first heard of Sarah, our child's birthmother, she was trying to decide whether or not to have an abortion, keep her child, or place him for adoption. At this point we could do nothing but wait for her decision; again we had no control and felt vulnerable.*

Our attorney called asking if we wanted to speak with Sarah and her mother on the phone. He would introduce us over a conference call and then allow us to talk privately. I have never felt so many butterflies, and a million fears surfaced within minutes: What if she didn't like us? What if we didn't like her? What would we talk about? After the initial hellos, there were laughter, tears, and a strong sense of love that I never would have thought possible between virtual strangers.

We all felt strongly that God had brought us together. That helped seal the bond that began that day and continues with each day of our child's life. We talked again a few days later and decided to meet. Sarah would fly up to spend several days with us in our home.

She made the trip when she was seven months pregnant. When she stepped off the plane, we embraced and then fumbled shyly with words while retrieving her luggage. We were in the car for about five minutes when she began to sing along with the radio and then giggled that she must not be nervous anymore. We all relaxed. We had a wonderful visit, a time for us to get acquainted that will always be fondly remembered. She was reassured about the home her child would be raised in; we were able to express our gratitude for her wonderful gift. When she left, we had agreed not to meet again before the birth. None of us knew if she would be able to go through with the adoption.

We left for her hometown the day the baby was due. Sarah had become more and more emotional, and we tried to brace ourselves for another disappointment. We met her parents, and this was another beautiful experience: They weren't much older than us! Her mother gave us a letter for the baby to read as an adult—a letter from Sarah explaining her reasons for the adoption, along with pictures of Sarah and her family to give our child some sense of his biological roots.

The day our son was born was truly one of mixed emotions. We were so happy for ourselves, but felt Sarah and her family's pain. We held him in our arms when he was 4 hours old and spent as much time at the hospital as they would allow. When we left, there were hugs, tears, and that same inexpressible love that we had felt before. Sarah did not look at her son at birth, but held him in her arms and said her goodbyes before she went home. When we left the hospital with that tiny bundle, we knew he was ours.

We have heard from Sarah twice since Kevin's birth: once when he was about a year old and again before his fourth birthday. I do feel fear when I see the envelope in the mail, but it is only fleeting because of the openness of our adoption. When we visited with Sarah we told her that the door would always be open to her. If she ever wanted to inquire about our son's health and happiness, we would reply. If it weren't for her, we wouldn't have our wonderful son. How could we deny her? She in turn assured us that she would never try to intrude and we trust her in that. Her letters were written to let us know that she is happy and to request some pictures, which we sent along with news of Kevin. Her sister has told us the pictures and letter have brought great comfort to Sarah.

Open adoption is relatively new, so it's hard to know how it will affect our children as they become adults. We discussed the possibility of Sarah meeting Kevin when he is an adult and have assured her that we would not be opposed to it if he chooses to do so. We do not feel threatened: We may not have given birth to him, but he is our son in every way and no one can ever take that away. Our love is too secure.

I think closed adoptions will soon be a thing of the past and the fears and myths will be put aside where they belong. By being sensitive to one another, expressing fears and expectations, and understanding each other, I believe that all members of the adoption triangle can emerge as happy and whole beings.

The concept of open adoption is a controversial one, sure to raise both vehement pro and con opinions. Some argue it is a vehicle to change traditionally negative adoption attitudes and methods and a healthier approach for all triad members. Others fear it will create confusion and further pain for all involved. Nonetheless, the practice has been growing in our society in reaction both to the closed records of past decades and to an increasing demand by birthmothers to know where their children will be placed.

In this arrangement the identities of both parties are known beforehand, and communication in some form may continue between the birthparents and the adoptive family after the child's adoption. Most often this involves an exchange of letters and pictures once or twice a year initially and then occasional correspondence as the child grows older. In a few cases visitation between the family and the birthparents also occurs. This is commonly referred to as "cooperative adoption." In any case these arrangements should be constantly examined and modified if appropriate.

Each of the adults involved must be mature and able to put the best interests of the child first. This is often painful. The birthmother may eagerly await pictures and news but fear blame or resentment when the child realizes that she relinquished him or her. Adoptive parents may also fear ongoing communication, a poignant and painful reminder of their child's origins and their infertility. It is, as one father stated, "the eternal price you pay for parenting." Others consider these letters as statements of love that their child will cherish. Many adoptive parents fear that cooperative or open adoption will evolve into a coparenting arrangement, where the birthparents will interfere with their family relationships or compete for their child's love and loyalty. The child's feelings and emotional maturity must also be weighed when considering this arrangement. Will an open or cooperative relationship be loving and secure or confusing and alarming?

This type of adoption is not appropriate or desirable in every case. There are loaded issues surrounding adoption that make this arrangement a difficult one to contemplate, and each triad must decide whether it is right for them. Those who are currently involved with open adoption are social pioneers; their experiences may largely determine the future of this arrangement.

► *We have two adopted children. We adopted our oldest, Ben, in a closed agency adoption. Our daughter, Sally, was adopted independently. We told Ben, at a very young age, that he was adopted. When he was about 3, I could see he was hurt and confused about this "phantom birthmother" who gave him up out of love but was not a real person he had met. I told him he might be able to meet her when he was 18. I knew by the look of confusion and pain on his face that this was the wrong solution.*

The adoption agency facilitated an exchange of letters between Ben's birthmother and our family. We all met face to face when he was about 4. He has had mixed feelings about Joan, his birthmother, but he has at least seen and spoken with her. He now has a real person in mind when he thinks about his birthmother—someone to direct his feelings toward.

We met Sally's biological mother before her birth. Afterward, we exchanged many letters and finally took Sally to meet her just last month. Sally is just a toddler and it's hard to say what she thinks. Neither children's birthfathers have met them yet.

We are leaving the lines of communication open between both sets of birthparents and our family. As my children grow up, their feelings and needs will largely determine the amount and kind of contact we will have.

I feel that knowing their birthparents will help my kids cope with adoption and its painful identity issues, especially during adolescence. I also think both adoption and infertility are parallel lifelong processes. By openly addressing one, I am acknowledging the other.

On With Your Lives!

An adoptive family learns to differentiate between the biological and social ancestry of their child. While the birthparents provide a genetic history, the adoptive family provides social ancestors and a sense of community. Creating a family album or scrapbook of pictures and relics of your child's social ancestors is a way to reinforce this bond for this and future generations.

You'll also educate those around you about adoption, just as you did with infertility. This includes everyone who touches your family's life: relatives, friends, teachers, neighbors, and coworkers. Tell them what hurts and helps; what is myth and what is not.

Finally, remember that you are a family in every sense of the word. Feel the pride and joy you so richly deserve and move ahead to the new triumphs and challenges awaiting you.

CHAPTER 18

Pregnancy

► *I called the lab. They said positive. I shrieked. I called back to make sure they had the right person. "Yes, they said, "positive."*
I asked, "How often are there false positives?"

About half the couples treated for infertility will become pregnant at least once, and most of these will successfully birth a child. A discussion of the complex physical, emotional, and psychological processes of pregnancy and birth are beyond the scope of this book. For readings on these topics see the selected bibliography.

This chapter focuses on the the psychological and emotional issues of pregnancy and parenting after infertility. It may seem odd to include such a discussion in this book. Most of us think that bearing a child will banish the specter of infertility. In fact pregnancy and childbirth don't always erase infertility scars and often raise sensitive issues of their own.

Pregnant at Last!

► *When I called the doctor's office, a voice I didn't recognize came on the line: "Mrs. James? The test is positive. Is that good news?"*
Laughing and crying, I said, "Yes, that is good news!"

After months or years of infertility, a positive pregnancy test often evokes a spectrum of emotions, sometimes in succession or even all at once!

► *I wanted to pull people off the street and shout, "I'm pregnant! After three years of surgery, drugs, charts, and buckets of tears, infertile me is pregnant!"*

Like marathon runners crossing the finish line, most infertile couples feel incredibly high when a pregnancy is confirmed: "At long last, we did it!" The good news is often greeted with screams, laughter, tears, and a delightful hysteria that may last for hours. When a pregnancy occurs after a poor prognosis for success, a previous miscarriage, or fertility surgery, it is indeed a sweet victory. Some want to shout their joy from the rooftops, call everyone they know, and openly rejoice. Other couples favor a quiet, private celebration. Whatever your inclination, savor and enjoy this moment.

After months or years of dashed hopes and disappointment, some react to their pregnancy with anxiety. They may fear a miscarriage, especially after a previous pregnancy loss. Others may be afraid that mother and/or baby will be harmed during pregnancy or birth, or that their present happiness just can't last.

► *Accepting this pregnancy has been a long drawn-out process accomplished in little steps week by week. Somewhere in the back of my head has lurked the idea that if I feel too secure in this baby, God or fate may snatch it cruelly away. I find myself reacting to all the normal anxieties threefold. Any deviation from the norm has been an opportunity to worry.*

You may seesaw between positive and negative feelings: excited that it's finally happened, yet frightened about what lies ahead. The confirmation of impending parenthood may also be a sobering notion. As one woman recalled:

► *One day it dawned on me: Not only was I pregnant, I was going to have a* baby! *After several years of infertility, I was more than prepared for pregnancy, but was I ready to be a mother?*

After functioning for so long in an infertile state of mind, many women are incredulous that they are actually pregnant. Once the news is out, and especially after your pregnancy begins to show, the world perceives and treats you very differently. Many people want to share and enjoy your happiness.

► *Being pregnant had been a fantasy for so long it was hard not to believe it wasn't still all in my head. My family wanted to talk baby showers, and I couldn't even talk pregnant yet. My mind seemed eternally on hold. I wasn't about to believe anything until I was past the time I had previously miscarried. Then I found myself thinking I'd wait to get excited after I had passed 12 weeks; then, after I felt the baby move. At six months I walked into a store and a clerk asked, "When is your baby due?" Surprised, my first thought was, "How in the world did she know I was expecting a baby?"*

There are no "right" reactions to pregnancy after infertility. Because you haven't followed the normal path to pregnancy, it is logical that you may react differently from women who achieve it easily. Try sharing your thoughts with other infertile women who have become pregnant. Hearing that they have similar reactions is calming.

► *Let it be known there are happiness and joy to be measured against those moments filled with anxiety and fear. There are days when I do feel the glowing picture of motherhood, days I want to shout aloud how beautiful I feel to be growing this baby at long last. And always it is worth the years it took to get here. It will not erase them; they will always be a part of me. But I can look forward and accept that this pregnancy starts a new time in my life with new battles to be won.*

Your pregnancy marks the end of primary infertility and the beginning of the transition into parenthood. You are both truly expecting a major life change that will bring new and challenging roles. Enjoy your pregnancy, from the first news to birth, as a poignant, exciting adventure.

Joining the Fertile World

► *I realize that there are problems common to both infertility and pregnancy to deal with. One was the feeling of being cut off from the very network of people who have been of support. On the other hand I found that when we announced our pregnancy to family and friends, suddenly an abundance of people wanted to share in the good news and bask in the excitement. It was difficult to deal with everyone being so positive. Where were they when the going was tough? When I needed to talk? When I was worried and depressed? Although their enthusiasm was genuine, it was easy to resent it so late in the game.*

After long-term infertility, it is common to experience a sort of identity crisis when you become pregnant. Although now a card-carrying member of the "prego club," you may still identify emotionally with infertility. Instead you will be entering a world of prenatal exercise and childbirth classes, mothers' groups, babysitting coops, preschools, and tot parks. Few of your new acquaintances can relate to your fertility problems.

You will also be showered with approval, interest, and support from friends, relatives, and the world at large. Many people smile warmly at your growing belly as they pass you on the street. At last you've arrived–a pregnant lady in a fertile world. This attention and change of identity can be disconcerting.

Remembering your own envy and awkwardness associated with pregnant friends or relatives, you understand why it is painful for your infertile friends to share your happiness. Now you are pregnant and, fearing a common bond is gone, may avoid contact with infertile acquaintances.

► *Every time I heard of a fellow infertile's pregnancy, I remember thinking, "Hurray, there's one for our side" and a feeling of hope would come over me. So when I learned I was pregnant, why did I sit in the back of our support group meeting, wringing my hands, heart pounding, afraid to share the good news? How could I tell all these people that I had something we all wanted so badly? I worried that this meant leaving a group of people I had learned to love and cherish for their never-ending support and encouragement. What would happen now that things had changed?*

An honest exchange of feelings is usually the best approach: a discussion often filled with tears, laughter, joy, and with envy. Many of these friendships will probably weather your pregnancy and continue afterward.

For a time you may feel you don't fit in either world. Accept these ambivalent feelings for now. Your pregnancy becomes more real as time passes, and with parenthood your horizons will expand as you meet people who don't fit the norms of our society: child-free couples, families with special children, single and adoptive parents, and those struggling with secondary infertility.

Changes During Pregnancy

► *Of course I had years of expectations saved for this momentous occasion. I was to be the glowing Madonna, wind in my hair, maternal smile on my lips. Instead, I have been tired, pimply, gaseous, crabby, and sick.*

► *Except for a little indigestion, I felt wonderful during my entire pregnancy. I loved being pregnant, enjoyed watching the baby grow and move, and felt productive in every area of my life.*

Every woman's pregnancy is different. During the next 40 weeks (more or less), your physical condition and feelings toward the pregnancy may vacillate or change. Some women look and feel wonderful, blessed with that proverbial Madonna glow. Many, though, experience nausea and other discomforts for two, three, or even six months. There is no way to predict whether this will happen to you.

A small percentage of women (whether formerly infertile or not) develop medical problems that affect their pregnancy. Such a development brings sadness, disbelief, or fear. It is important to realize that these feelings are common to *all* pregnant women.

► *My last trimester was quite stressful. I had frequent ultrasounds to check the baby's growth and monitor a uterine problem. I was grateful to be pregnant, of course, but I was also confused and frightened by this unexpected "problem" pregnancy.*

The initial delight with your pregnancy may fade, especially if physical discomfort or complications persist. Many formerly infertile women, however, are reluctant to complain, even if they are sick or miserable for months! As one woman remarked, "After all, hadn't I always envied that look of nausea on other women's faces?" Give yourself the luxury of complaining just like most pregnant women do.

The Couple's Relationship

► *The hardest thing to accept has been that this would not be the pregnancy I had wished for and imagined for so many years. I could never breeze through this, like those women who got pregnant easily or accidentally, and act as if nothing dramatic was taking place. In my second month I made the dreadful mistake of running (horrors!) to meet my husband, only to find him furious with me for taking such a "chance." This pregnancy was too precious for us to take nonchalantly.*

Many infertile couples find it difficult to relax and enjoy their pregnancy. This feat took so long to accomplish, at such a high emotional and perhaps physical price, that they worry endlessly. What if something goes wrong and they miscarry? They may never have another chance. Months of tension may follow.

Real life, with its inevitable pressures and problems, soon comes sharply back into focus. After a few months of pregnancy, some couples are surprised that their pregnancy hasn't brought complete happiness into their lives. They still have bad days, arguments, and other new pressures.

► *For all the times I have said to myself, "If only I were pregnant," this long-sought pregnancy has yet to pay the bills, remodel our living room, or change the weather. Life still goes on. Reality could never live up to the idyllic scene I had painted for myself.*

Genetic Testing

Our era of advanced technology offers a number of prenatal tests, such as amniocentesis and alpha fetoprotein blood analysis, which detect some genetic problems and birth defects. Because many couples are in their late twenties or early thirties when fertility problems are detected and treated, they are often 35 or older when they do conceive. As some genetic problems occur more often in older mothers, pregnant women over age 35 are often advised to undergo some of these tests.

In deciding whether to take genetic tests, both partners must assess the risks and advantages and their feelings about therapeutic abortion if a problem is detected. A woman undergoing amniocentesis, for example, runs a 1 in 200 to 300 chance (statistics vary among testing centers) of miscarrying as a result of the procedure. Genetic testing is a frightening experience for many couples, especially those who have waited years to conceive. They must weigh the testing risks against their probability of conceiving again.

Parenting after Infertility

► *I'm exhausted. I can't get anything done during the day because my son insists on being held and rocked. My dishes and laundry are piled up. I long for just 15 minutes to call my own and a hot cup of coffee.*

Still, all of this is much easier to bear than three days of infertility. As I rock, I think about what makes infertility so different from other life problems.

Now that I'm a parent I have met dozens of people who empathize with me. It seems everyone knows what it's like to be up all night with a crying baby. All I need to do is reach out and there are friends and family saying, "We've been there ourselves, you'll make it through." That is the difference between now and then. Where was all that support and understanding before? I faced my infertility on my own. It was, and still is, the most isolating, lonely, frustrating experience I have ever had.

► *Melinda is precious to us, and we are grateful for her presence. But yes, parenthood does wear thin at times. I struggle to juggle motherhood with my own pursuits of teaching and writing. But still feelings linger that fertiles don't understand. Each night I watch her sleep and recall the terrible childless years. I am humbled by, and grateful for, my miracle.*

Many parents are awed and overwhelmed by the miracle of their newborn. They also encounter months of sleepless nights, frazzled nerves, and tremendous personal and marital adjustment. A history of infertility does not exempt you from the chaos of early parenthood.

Now it's your wailing offspring, rather than the pain of being childless, that keeps you awake at night. Few first-time parents are accustomed to being on 24-hour call by a self-centered, crying infant—a helpless bundle who can't say what's wrong so you can fix it and go back to sleep. Older parents are especially tired by nighttime feedings. By the fifth or sixth week of round-the-clock duty and overall exhaustion, you may forget your own name and the fact that you actually struggled for this opportunity! Fortunately most kids eventually sleep through the night (until they're teenagers), colic recedes, and life again takes on a schedule.

Our infertility experience teaches us how fragile and tenuous life is, and that the conception, gestation, and birth of an infant is indeed a miracle. Perhaps we treasure our children in a different way from those who conceive easily. Without medical help and a great deal of luck, we would have missed this experience, and few of us ever forget that. This is perhaps the only reward of an infertility struggle: From the moment of your baby's birth, you have the wisdom that you have been given a precious and irreplacable gift: a child to love, treasure, and enjoy.

Each developmental stage—talking, crawling, walking, cutting and losing baby teeth, going off to nursery school and then kindergarten—is wonderful, amazing, and often bittersweet. We're aware of how soon our child will grow up, how we might not have another chance to parent, and how long we waited.

Leaving Infertility Behind?

► *You'd think that now that our vivacious, handsome little 2-year-old son is bounding about our house that those infertile feelings would never creep into our lives again. Well, believe me, they do. Amidst all our joy and happiness, a part of us still grieves about our infertility and for all those sad couples out there, especially those afraid to share their burden. Our experience of infertility helped shape who we are today.*

"Well, you've had a baby. It must be a relief that your infertility is finally over." This is a common observation after the birth of your child. We assume that pregnancy and parenthood will cure infertility, and for some this is probably true. After their child's birth, they count their blessings, content to be a family of three.

Others still feel infertile. One or both partners may yearn for another child, feeling that their family is not yet complete. Family planning becomes a confusing, somewhat ironic issue. Should they assume fertility and try for the ideal two- to four-year spacing between children? Or should they not use contraception and hope a pregnancy happens in due time? Some have tried this approach, and found themselves with two children 12 or 15 months apart—not an easy experience.

Some couples, unable to conceive a second time, must undergo yet another workup and treatment program. Familiar stresses resurface, as well as new ones unique to secondary infertility (see Chapter 6).

CHAPTER 19

Surrogate Mothers

► *Nancy, a wife and mother of two, felt a great deal of empathy for infertile men and women. Her own two kids meant so much to her that she could not imagine going through life without children. Whenever she read or heard about an infertile couple who desperately wanted a child, her heart went out to them.*

She conceived easily and both her pregnancies had been healthy with normal deliveries. For more than a year, Nancy thought about becoming a surrogate mother. She felt she would be able to detach herself from such a pregnancy and "give" the baby to the "real parents" at birth. She discussed her feelings with her husband and, although he didn't want any more children, he was supportive of a surrogate arrangement. She also spoke with her clergyman about her motivation to give the gift of life to a childless couple. He, too, lent his emotional support.

Nancy made her decision and, after several referrals, found a reputable adoption attorney who facilitated surrogate arrangements. At their first meeting she told him why she wanted to be a surrogate mother. They spoke at length about the legal, psychological, and ethical issues of a surrogate arrangement, and he explained the current California law, which held that children fathered by artificial insemination not performed by a physician were considered the biological children of the donor. Nancy then filled out a detailed questionnaire concerning her family history and health background. She told the attorney that she wanted to meet any interested couples, rather than bear a child for anonymous people she would never see. He, too, felt that all parties should meet beforehand to share their feelings and expectations.

Several months later, the attorney called her. An infertile couple, Sandy and Wes, wanted to meet her and discuss a surrogate arrangement. Everyone was nervous at first, but as they shared their respective feelings about infertility, each of them relaxed and began to hope that the arrangement would work.

The attorney then explained that he handled surrogate arrangements as "adoptions planned in advance." He followed the basic legal guidelines of independent adoption: like a birthmother, the surrogate was paid only reasonable medical, living, and counseling expenses. No "fee" would be paid to her for her surrogate "services." Nancy could, of course, work during the pregnancy if she chose; her employment would not affect payment for the agreed living, medical, and counseling expenses.

They also discussed contingencies if Nancy should miscarry or bear a child with a physical or mental handicap. Although the attorney could draw up a declaration of intent specifying these contingency agreements, he told them it would not be enforceable in court. They would have to trust each other on these points. He could, however, draw up a legally enforceable contract specifying a monthly allotment for allowable expenses once Nancy became pregnant.

Everyone agreed to think it over and meet again in one week. At their next meeting, they agreed to a surrogate arrangement and both the declaration of intent and a contract regarding payment of expenses were drawn up. Nancy would be paid $925 per month for living and counseling expenses, disbursed by the attorney in ten monthly installments. If she miscarried, she agreed to try insemination for another three cycles; if she became pregnant, any payments already received would be applied toward the second pregnancy. Sandy and Wes would pay for all legal expenses and any medical costs not covered by Nancy's medical insurance.

Nancy went through three inseminations before becoming pregnant. Sandy was disappointed with the first two failures, as if she herself were trying to get pregnant. During this time Sandy also vacillated between feelings of hope and excitement and sexual jealousy and inadequacy. Wes was excited about the idea of becoming a father but also concerned about Sandy's feelings.

From the first day Nancy felt a kind of emotional detachment about the baby. Although she loved the infant, she felt this was Sandy and Wes's baby; she was simply carrying it for them. She told both her children about the baby and that she was doing this to help a couple who couldn't have a child. With her husband's approval, Nancy also told their friends and family that she was a surrogate mother. Reactions ranged from shock and disapproval to that of her father, who said, "Bless you."

Sandy and Wes called her often during the pregnancy to see how she was doing. Nancy decided she would not see the baby after leaving the hospital. Some surrogates stay in touch with the couple after the birth of the baby, but Nancy thought that her role should end with the birth.

Nancy delivered a healthy seven pound, three ounce boy. Sandy and Wes were with her in the delivery room. When the baby was born, everyone cried, and Sandy said to her, "Thank you for giving us our lives."

Before Sandy and Wes took the baby home, Nancy spent some time alone with him in the hospital room. She said her heartfelt goodbyes and wished him a wonderful life. Her two children also came to see the baby to say hello and goodbye. Afterward Nancy lay thinking about that family's happiness and a flood of tears broke. Looking back, she says she did not cry because she longed for the baby, but because being a surrogate mother is so emotionally intense. Nancy later wrote a letter to the baby explaining what she did and why.

The baby will always hold a very special place in Nancy's heart, and she is proud of the gift she has given. She did work during the pregnancy and has saved that money for her children's educations.

Nancy realizes that many people will never understand why she became a surrogate mother in the first place, and why she didn't demand a large fee in the second. She thinks that if these people spent an hour with an infertile couple who desperately want a child, they would understand.

Surrogate mothers are women who contract with an infertile couple to undergo insemination with the husband's sperm, bear his biological child, and relinquish the baby to the couple. Single men also sometimes contract with a surrogate to bear a child. Variations of in vitro fertilization can also involve surrogate mothers. For example, a husband's or donor's sperm can be combined with an infertile woman's ova and implanted in a surrogate's womb.

To date about 600 babies have been born through surrogate arrangements in the United States. With the increasing incidence of infertility and a growing scarcity of adoptable infants, more couples in the future may consider enlarging their family in this way.

Like artificial insemination by donor (AID), a surrogate arrangement is a controversial infertility resolution and raises many of the same psychological and ethical issues as AID and adoption. The couple involves a third party to bear the husband's biological child, whom the wife will adopt. As with adoption, the surrogate's involvement is highly personal; she will carry a pregnancy to term and then birth and relinquish a child. Unlike AID and some types of adoption, however, the identity of the donor is known. She may meet the prospective parents and perhaps continue contact during her pregnancy; the couple may even attend the birth.

Surrogate arrangements often work out quite well. The couple and surrogate mother may meet, like one another, and form a relationship of mutual respect. In rare cases the surrogate mother stays in contact with the family.

On the other hand some infertile couples have reported difficult, painful experiences with surrogate arrangements. Some have invested substantial amounts of emotional and financial resources only to have the birthmother "take back," or refuse to relinquish the child.

Deciding on a Surrogate Arrangement

Many attorneys, therapists, physicians, and ethicists are concerned that an infertile couple is especially vulnerable to financial and emotional exploitation. It is sometimes difficult, under the emotional stress of infertility, to weigh the risks and advantages of a surrogate arrangement.

Carefully consider the many factors involved in this decision. A first step may be to examine, as individuals and as a couple, your feelings about these difficult issues:

- Are you both comfortable with having another woman bear the husband's biological child?
- Is this the best infertility resolution for the both of you?
- Have you thought about genetic or psychological screening for the surrogate? Will you ask her to have an amniocentesis or other test for birth defects? What if such testing reveals a problem?
- In case of miscarriage will you ask the surrogate to try insemination again?

- Can you afford the expense of a surrogate arrangement?
- What will you do if the child is born with a mental or physical handicap?
- Will you tell your child about the surrogate mother? Will you keep in contact with her? Have you considered search issues as your child grows up?

Contracting with a surrogate is also a legal gamble. The couple will have to trust that she will fulfill her part of the bargain: refrain from intercourse with other men during insemination to assure paternity, maintain a healthy pregnancy and seek adequate prenatal care, and relinquish the baby at birth.

A couple considering this arrangement will need considerable financial resources: usually at least $12,000 and often more. This money is considered a gift and cannot be recovered if the arrangement falls through.

Finding a Surrogate

If, after considering these issues, a couple opts for a surrogate arrangement, their next step is to find a suitable surrogate and reach a mutual agreement. Some couples search for themselves by advertising in newspapers or magazines for a woman willing to bear a child for a fee plus expenses. Others seek a reputable adoption attorney who also facilitates surrogate arrangements. Such attorneys are often approached by potential surrogates and may make introductions. In addition a growing number of agencies, usually run by a staff of attorneys, psychologists, and perhaps social workers, match surrogates with infertile couples or individuals.

The procedures, fees, ethical standards, and reputation of both attorneys and surrogate agencies varies considerably. Before consenting to any arrangement or paying any fees, carefully research the reputation and methods of the agency or lawyer. To ensure that they employ competent staff and operate within the law, check with their county's district attorney's office.

Once a potential surrogate is found, the couple may meet with her to negotiate a contract, or an agency may match the parties and facilitate communication or arrange a meeting. Many experts suggest that the surrogate mother receive counseling or psychiatric evaluation to ensure that she is willing and able to give up the child after birth. This is not a guarantee, however, that she actually will.

Cost

Expenses for a surrogate arrangement vary widely. Costs for an arrangement similar to that of our case study would include $9,250, paid in ten equal monthly installments, for living and counseling costs for the surrogate, and perhaps an additional $2000 for legal fees. Any medical expenses not covered by the surrogate's insurance would also be added. Because Nancy had medical coverage, this arrangement cost the couple $11,250; the cost would have been higher if they had been responsible for the delivery and hospital stay. Note that in our example, Nancy was not paid a fee for her surrogate services. Such an arrangement follows the financial guidelines of private adoption. One attorney, who has facilitated both independent adoptions and surrogate arrangements, likens this approach to an "adoption planned in advance."

Many surrogate agencies, however, include a fee for "surrogate services," usually ranging from $10,000 to $15,000 or more in addition to the other expenses. In these cases the couple's total cost often exceeds $20,000. Carefully investigate any program that charges large sums of money for "surrogate services" or unidentified expenses.

In any event monies paid to surrogates are considered gifts, regardless of whether a child is conceived or born. Advance fees to agencies may also be forfeited.

Legal Issues

If the parties agree to mutually satisfactory terms and fees, two written agreements are usually prepared and signed by both. The first is a statement of the intent of the parties to enter into this relationship and contingencies for such occurrences as miscarriage or birth defects. Such an agreement is based solely on trust; *it is not enforceable in a court of law.*

Either party may discontinue the arrangement; only under extraordinary circumstances, if at all, can the birthmother be legally ordered to surrender the child. If she should want to keep the child, some states would hold the biological father responsible for child support payments. In California, for example, donors at one time had no claim to paternity of children conceived through artificial insemination of their sperm. The California appellate court has recently ruled that any child conceived by artificial insemination that was *not* performed in a physician's office is the biological child of the donor (*Jhordan C. v. Mary K.* (1986) 179 CA3d 386). In light of this ruling, some attorneys and surrogate agencies now advise that inseminations be done by someone other than a physician, thus establishing the donor's rights to paternity. It remains to be seen whether the appellate court's ruling will be upheld in California, or if other states will adopt this interpretation.

The second agreement is often a legally enforceable contract specifying and itemizing acceptable living, medical, and counseling costs. Fees for legal and administrative costs, as well as charges of $10,000 or more for the "services" of the birthmother may also be included in this contract.

Note that there are vague distinctions between an illegal or black market adoption and paying large amounts of money for "living" or "miscellaneous" expenses or "services" to a surrogate. *Couples considering a surrogate arrangement are strongly urged to seek legal counsel from a reputable attorney, with no vested interest in this contractual relationship, who knows about surrogate and adoption laws in all states involved.*

Psychological and Ethical Issues

Like AID, a surrogate arrangement raises several complex psychological and ethical issues.

For the Surrogate

Many in our society consider surrogate mothering immoral or emotionally and physically exploitive of the birthmother. They question whether a woman can truly give away this baby without permanent emotional damage. Indeed some surrogates underestimate the emotional and psychological impact of this experience. After birthing and relinquishing the child, they may feel depressed or even grief-stricken. Other surrogates feel fulfillment and joy in giving the gift of life to a couple or individual unable to birth a child. They are able to separate themselves emotionally from the pregnancy and child.

Some people regard the insemination a thin guise for adultery. A single woman may be viewed as immoral for participating in this process. If the surrogate is married, she often hears similar criticism from family, friends, and acquaintances.

For the Infertile Couple

When the couple decides to resolve their problem through a surrogate arrangement, several issues may surface for them both as a couple and as individuals.

They may encounter sexual problems similar to those of couples going through AID. In surrogate arrangements, it is usually the infertile wife who feels inadequate and perhaps sexually jealous. Her husband's sperm is being inseminated into another woman—a fertile one yet! Some women who are not clinically sterile may also fantasize that they could still become pregnant.

Their sex life may also be partially controlled by the surrogate's menstrual cycle. To ensure sperm that are optimally fertile they may have to refrain from intercourse a day or two before inseminations. This is a poignant reminder of both her infertility and their inability to bear a child as a couple.

Both partners may be excited and hopeful about becoming parents at last. Many couples are so tired of their infertility that they welcome this resolution as a closure. Some infertile wives take an active role in the medical and legal planning of this arrangement and report that they are relieved and happy to move forward with their lives.

The fact remains that this will be the husband's biological child. Many men are excited about fathering a child at last and again feel in control of their lives. Their wives may share this happiness yet also find this a sad and lonely time. They may grieve for their loss of a genetic lineage and, unlike their husbands, experience the doubts and stresses of an adoptive parent-to-be. These differing perspectives can cause misunderstanding and division between the couple.

For the Family

Like the AID family, those who parent through a surrogate arrangement face unique and painful issues. They must decide if and when to tell their child about the surrogate mother and what role, if any, she will have in their lives. In later years their child may wish to search for her, and vice versa.

In addition the family must decide what to tell their family and friends about their child. They cannot, as they could with an AID situation, pretend that this is the couple's pregnancy. The wife is not pregnant. They will have to tell others about the surrogate or simply say their child is adopted and omit the fact of the husband's paternity.

Coping Suggestions

- Seek legal and medical information, emotional support, and psychological counseling from qualified professionals about surrogate arrangements and their unique issues. (It is wise for the birthmother to do this also.) These contacts can be helpful during the decision-making process, inseminations, and pregnancy and after the child's birth.

- Since insemination times can be emotionally and sexually difficult for an infertile couple, try to express love for each other in different ways: long talks, walks, romantic dinners, touching, and holding. Expressions of humor, patience, and love toward each other help a lot.
- Decide how much information about this arrangement to share with others, and devise a script to use when asked about the circumstances of your child's birth.
- Accept this unique method of enlarging your family as a lifelong process. Some issues about your infertility as a couple, or the surrogate's role in your lives, will probably surface periodically over the years.

CHAPTER 20

Child-Free Living

► *My fantasies of motherhood had soft rosy edges that four or five hours of being with real-life children quickly dispelled. It made it easier to enjoy the parts of my day that were there precisely because I had no children. People with small children don't have the luxuries of time with their spouses, leisurely dinners, spur-of-the-moment shopping trips, or the quiet to curl up with a good book or even the newspaper! It was nice to remember that all the advantages were not on one side; both life-styles have their pros and cons.*

Traditionally the term *childlessness* has been used to describe a life-style without biological or adopted children. Until recently couples without children accepted society's notion that their lives were empty, boring, unhappy, and less than fulfilled. This stereotype is now being challenged and a new term, *child-free living,* better describes the decision not to parent. This option, a valid and viable resolution to infertility, can lead to a happy, positive, and enriching life-style.

Couples choose a child-free life-style for a variety of reasons. Some may be fertile but believe it is irresponsible to reproduce at this time. They view our planet as dangerously overcrowded, with pollution and nuclear war threatening the quality of life. Others regard childrearing as expensive, time-consuming, and stressful—an experience for which they are not suited.

Many infertile couples also consider this option when biological parenthood seems unlikely. Those who attach great importance to pregnancy and birth often opt for child-free living rather than adoption.

Making the Choice

► *I had an ectopic pregnancy six years ago and haven't been able to conceive since. Both my husband and I wanted to experience pregnancy and birth. We have also both witnessed painful adoption experiences among our families. After lengthy grieving we've opted for child-free living. And I can now say, "Yes! We are happy and still very much in love!"*

Once we decide to have a child, most of us assume pregnancy will "just happen." After repeated pregnancy losses or a medical diagnosis of infertility, many infertile couples look for a way to solve their dilemma. In some respects child-free living is the most difficult choice among the options. Unlike birthing or adopting a child, the child-free option is usually *revocable* for some time. You can change your mind tomorrow, next month, or perhaps several years from now and pursue further medical treatment or adoption. The possibility of reversing this choice can make the decision-making process even more perplexing.

There are several variations of the child-free choice: a permanent decision to stop trying for pregnancy altogether (perhaps one partner even undergoing sterilization to remove the pressure of infertility), letting Nature take its course and remaining child-free if pregnancy does not occur, or a temporary child-free life-style while long-range goals and resolutions are considered.

Couples usually begin weighing the child-free option by reassessing their original motivation to become pregnant. Some consider biological parenthood an important life achievement and want to experience pregnancy and birth. Others assume they are expected to reproduce by their families and society. Some look to offspring to care for them in illness and old age or to continue their lineage.

Once they define their motivation, the couple must grapple with the myths surrounding this option:

- Life is empty and meaningless without children.
- Those who do not parent will be immersed in grief and regrets forever.
- A child-free life ends with isolation and abandonment in old age.

Having overcome these myths, child-free couples realize that having children does not guarantee a perfect, happy life. There is no reason to assume that your children will reproduce themselves, care for you in your old age, or even invite you to Thanksgiving dinner! Still there may be moments of remorse and regret. It is important to remember that *all* major life decisions are questioned and reevaluated at some time. A better perspective might be, "Make the choice that you will regret the least!" One woman spoke wistfully of "not being anybody's Mommy." Although saddened by this reality, she also saw its positive side. She now had to develop her own identity and interests.

Through honest, direct, and frequent communication, some couples quickly reach agreement on a child-free life-style. For others, the decision-making process may be a long and painful one. In some cases one spouse favors adoption while the other leans toward child-free living. During such disagreement a couple may feel angry and isolated and fear they are drifting apart. Perhaps the fight against infertility has been a central focus for years and has forged a bond between them. Although it is a relief in one sense, abandoning the struggle can also be disorienting and threatening. A couple may wonder what will hold them together after their infertility is resolved.

To avoid an impasse the couple must complete grieving for their lost fertility, work together toward compromise, and reshape future goals. During this difficult time it is important to remember that you can become close again. Once a resolution is chosen, many couples report a return of energy, enthusiasm, and control of their lives.

Social and Family Pressures

► *It was difficult for my mother to accept my decision. She raised six children and now all her friends were grandmothers. She wanted grandchildren of her own.*

► *Strangers will ask, "Any children?" I say, "No." There is usually a silence and then, "Oh." The nosier ones will ask why not. If you state you have a fertility problem, they want to treat you and tell you all the cures. I've learned to educate them.*

One woman observed that while the decision to adopt is usually supported and approved by one's family, a child-free choice is often a lonely and contested one. Your decision may evoke criticism, anger, and pressure to adopt from family and friends. It may seem as if you're reliving your initial infertility struggle.

Once you make your choice, refrain from arguing or defending it to others. Rehashing your decision is exhausting, frustrating, and unnecessary, because most fertile people won't understand or empathize with your situation. Don't feel you have to defend your child-free choice or argue its merits: You owe no one any apologies or explanations.

With time social pressures subside as family and friends accept your decision. As your peer group ages and their children grow up, there will also be less focus on pregnancy, birth, and parenting in your daily life. In fact some child-free couples later find themselves supporting friends and relatives when their children leave home. The "empty nest syndrome" can be similar to the loneliness of infertility.

Making Children a Part of Your Life

► *A very special friend put her baby in my arms and left us alone. I cuddled that infant and fell in love. That child and I have had a special relationship ever since.*

► *I was furious when my younger sister got pregnant. My mother's delight was very painful to see. But I have faced my envy and now love my role as Auntie. I dote on my nieces and nephews and then give them back!*

Your child-free life-style should not isolate you from the joy and special company of children. There are children everywhere and countless ways to include them in your daily activities. Nephews, nieces, cousins, and friends' children enjoy spending time with fun-loving adults. Outings to the playground, zoo, swimming pool, circus, theater, or amusement park create wonderful memories for you and the kids and a welcome respite for Mom and Dad.

Local schools and churches welcome volunteers to work with kids. Perhaps you have a special talent in music, woodworking, cooking, art, computers, or fishing to share. Many local kids' softball, football, and soccer teams need volunteer coaches and organizers. Scouting organizations, Big Brother and Big Sister programs, local YMCAs and YWCAs, tutoring services, and programs for troubled youngsters also need volunteers.

Coping Suggestions

- Allow yourselves to grieve thoroughly the loss of your fertility. This loss must be acknowledged and grieved by *both* of you. Although each person mourns in his or her own time, periods of six months to a year are common. See Chapter 1 for more discussion of this process and coping suggestions.
- Find emotional support.

► *Our first infertility support group meeting heavily emphasized adoption. I left thinking, "That's how they fix infertility. Adoption must be the only cure and solution."*

Later we drifted away from the group. Adoption just wasn't the answer for us.

Infertile couples soon discover that most emotional support is geared toward achieving pregnancy or adoption. In fact the child-free choice is often a taboo subject. Couples who consider or select this option often feel outnumbered, overwhelmed, or even ostracized by those favoring adoption, AID, in vitro fertilization, or other alternatives.

Resource organizations that provide support for a child-free life-style are listed in Appendix A. RESOLVE can also refer you to other couples who have chosen this resolution.

- Develop an extended family network of friends and relatives. It is important to have a sense of community. Seek out others you admire and enjoy. Include those with and without children, single folks, and those older and younger than yourselves. Many of your relatives, church friends, working colleagues, and neighbors are eager for friendship and company.
- Celebrate your decision. You may be the only ones enthusiastic about your choice at first. Celebrate this rite of passage with a special vacation, adventure, or renewal of your commitment to each other. This is also an opportunity to reshape your future as individuals and a couple. Reconsider educational and career goals, as well as hobbies and volunteer work.
- Enjoy your child-free life. Enjoy the luxuries that come with child-free living. Travel, sleep late, indulge in spur-of-the-moment impulses and outings. This is also an opportunity to develop your own interests and enrich your marriage. Child-free couples are able to spend lots of time together. Enjoy and treasure your special mate!

- Acknowledge your family of two. Every couple begins their relationship as a family of two. Regardless of whether you raise children, you will greet old age as a twosome again. The experience of infertility can strengthen your family and provide wisdom and understanding for the challenges that lie ahead.

  You *are,* and *will continue to be,* a family of two! Keep scrapbooks, photo albums, and journals of your travels and adventures. Create holiday traditions and special birthday and anniversary rituals to celebrate your unique and loving family.

EPILOGUE

Some Lessons Learned

Even though I had birthed a baby, I believed I would live with the identity and grief of being secondarily infertile for the rest of my life. Rereading my journals of the last decade, I see that my healing was a slow, painstaking process of acceptance and reconciliation. I also recognize a few milestones that marked my progress. One was the recognition that it was time to stop the medical treatments—and finding the courage to do so. Another was Bob's and my acceptance of our infertility and reaffirmation of our commitment to each other. Perhaps the most important was my change of identity from a defeated, immobilized infertile "victim" to a healthy, productive, and self-respecting writer, wife, and mother who'd had fertility problems.

With these changes, accomplished gradually over nearly a decade, came a relocation of my sadness, pain, and grief. These feelings have drifted into small pockets within my heart and know their place. No longer obsessions or raw wounds, they have healed and been absorbed into my history like the scars from my surgeries—reminders that I am permanently changed. Because they no longer threaten my spirit or consume my thoughts, they are free to surface when I recall a trip to the operating room or when I listen to the heartache of an infertile friend.

I had healed to this point when I submitted my final manuscript to my publisher. A month later I became pregnant with my second child—an incredibly lucky and truly unexpected gift for a couple who had gently put that dream aside. This miracle has allowed me finally to join the other 85 percent of humanity who conceive a baby the "normal" way—without tests, treatments, drugs, or surgery—and to complete the family we had imagined. At long last I've found my children and brought them into this world.

I am sadly aware that not all infertile couples experience a pregnancy and that my present perceptions are influenced by my recent good fortune. Still I believe that the closure of my infertility began, not with either of my pregnancies, but with my acceptance of my limitations and determination to realize my potential despite them. At that point I left behind the label, identity, and crutch of infertility. It was time to stand or fall on my own character and achievements.

Looking back, I can't say I'm glad that infertility happened to me or that I would ever choose to strengthen myself with such a painful challenge. I can say that a lot of good has come from the experience. I have made lifelong friends who have loved, encouraged, and inspired me by their examples. Bob and I have learned what matters most in our lives—our marriage, children, and those who support and nurture us. And we have been afforded a rare opportunity to understand the fragility of life and the healing power of love, communion, and empathy between people.

Perhaps this is the reward at the end of an infertility struggle: the wisdom, acquired at a fairly young age, of what indeed matters to you.

Glossary
Bibliography
Appendixes
Index

GLOSSARY

abortion The termination of a pregnancy, initiated either spontaneously by the body or intentionally by medical intervention.

abruptio placentae A condition in which the placenta separates from the uterus.

acrosin An enzyme contained in the sperm head that helps the sperm penetrate the ova.

acrosome A cap enclosed in the head of the sperm, which contains enzymes that aid in fertilization.

ACTH *See* adrenocorticotropic hormone.

acute salpingitis Inflammation of the Fallopian tube caused by an infection.

adenoma A small benign tumor.

adhesions Scar tissue formed by the body after surgery, disease, infection, or inflammation.

adnexa The ovaries and Fallopian tubes.

adoption An arrangement, sanctioned by legal decree, in which an individual or couple parents and raises the biological child of others.

adoption triad The three parties involved in any adoption: the birthparents, the adoptive parents, and the adopted child (adoptee).

adrenocorticotropic hormone (ACTH) A hormone produced by the pituitary, which stimulates the adrenal glands to release cortisol hormone.

agglutinization The clumping of two or more sperm together.

AID *See* artificial insemination by donor.

AIH *See* artificial insemination by husband.

amenorrhea The absence of menstrual cycles.

amenorrhea galactorrhea The absence of menstrual cycles along with the presence of milk in the breasts.

amniocentesis A test done during pregnancy (often in women over 35 years of age), which examines amniotic fluid for chromosomal characteristics.

ampulla The middle section of the Fallopian tube.

androgens Male hormones produced by both sexes.

andrologist A urologist who specializes in male reproductive problems.

andrology The study of the male reproductive system.

anesthesia The numbing of pain through drugs.

anovulation The absence of ovulation.

anoxia An absence or deficiency of oxygen which may affect the fetus during labor or birth.

artificial insemination by donor (AID) A process in which sperm from a donor male is inseminated in a fertile woman in the hope of conception and successful pregnancy.

artificial insemination by husband (AIH) A process in which the sperm of a husband is inseminated into his mate's vagina, cervix, or uterus.

asthenospermia A condition in which less than half the sperm in the ejaculate are motile.

atretic process A natural process in which most of the immature oocytes a female is born with slowly disintegrate during her childhood and reproductive years.

azoospermia A total absence of sperm in the ejaculate.

basal body temperature (BBT) chart A chart used to graph daily basal (upon awakening and before any activity) body temperature during the menstrual cycle.

bicornate uterus A physical abnormality of the uterus in which it is divided partially or totally by a tissue membrane (septum), sometimes found in women whose mothers took DES during their pregnancies.

birth control pills Synthetic female hormones used as contraceptives and/or in treatment of such disorders as endometriosis.

birthparents The biological parents of an adopted child.

bovine cervical mucus test A male infertility test that checks the sperm's ability to penetrate cervical mucus.

bromocriptine (Parlodel) A drug that inhibits prolactin hormone secretion.

capacitation A process occurring after ejaculation that alters the sperm so it can penetrate an egg.

CAT scan An X-ray technique that produces a computerized picture of the interior of the body.

caudal anesthesia A type of anesthetic that is injected into the air spaces around the spinal column and numbs the nerve endings leading to the legs and pelvic area.

cervical mucus Secretions of the cervix, which usually change character throughout the menstrual cycle and are responsible for sperm transport, storage, and filtering.

cervix The narrow opening (or neck) that connects the uterus to the vagina; able to dilate many times its size during labor and delivery.

cesarean birth The delivery of a baby through an abdominal incision rather than vaginally.

child-free living A resolution to infertility in which the couple opts for a life-style without parenting, either temporarily or permanently.

chlamydia A sexually transmitted disease that may cause impaired fertility or sterility.

chocolate cysts Ovarian cysts formed by endometriosis; also called endometriomas.

chromosome The parts of the nucleus of a body cell that hold the parent's genetic information in twisted strands of a substance called deoxyribonucleic acid (DNA).

chronic salpingitis The tubal scarring or blockages caused by infection.

cilia The hairlike projections in the Fallopian tubes that propel the ovum toward the uterus.

climacteric The gradual cessation of menses, usually occurring between the ages of 40 and 50, that culminates in a final period (the menopause).

clitoris A female sexual organ composed of erectile tissue and highly sensitive to stimulation.

clomiphene citrate (Serophene or Clomid) A commonly prescribed "fertility drug" that induces ovulation.

complete abortion Expulsion of all fetal and placental tissue by the body.

conception The fertilization of an ovum by a sperm.

corpus luteum The body that forms on the ovary after the follicle has ovulated; secretes progesterone hormone.

cumulus oophorus The cloudlike outer covering of the ovum.

curettage Scraping of the uterine lining.

danazol (Danocrine) A drug derived from male hormones used to treat endometriosis.

DES *See* diethylstilbestrol.

dextran A slippery substance sometimes placed in the abdominal cavity during pelvic surgery to inhibit scarring.

diethylstilbestrol (DES) A synthetic form of estrogen given to some pregnant women between 1940 and 1971 to prevent miscarriage; sometimes caused abnormalities in their offspring.

dilation and curettage (D and C) A medical procedure, done under anesthesia, that scrapes the interior of the uterus.

duct obstruction A blockage in the epididymis or vas deferens of the male.

dysmenorrhea Painful menses.

ectopic pregnancy A pregnancy that implants outside the uterus, usually in the Fallopian tube, and creates a life threatening condition.

ejaculate Semen discharged through the urethra during male climax.

electrosurgery A microsurgery technique that uses electrical needles for cutting or adhesion removal.

embryo A term used to describe the fertilized ovum through about the eighth week of pregnancy.

endocrine system A group of glands that contribute hormones to the bloodstream.

endocrinologist A physician who specializes in problems of the endocrine system.

endometrial biopsy A female workup procedure in which a bit of endometrial lining is scraped or suctioned and then tested for maturation.

endometriomas Ovarian cysts formed by endometriosis.

endometriosis A condition in which the endometrial cells that normally line the uterus travel to other sites, implant, and grow during the menstrual cycle.

endometrium The lining of the uterus, which nurtures the fertilized embryo or is expelled during menstruation.

epididymis The duct system that transports the sperm and is the place where they mature and develop the ability to fertilize.

epididymitis Inflammation of the epididymis duct.

epididymovasotomy Surgery to remedy a blockage within the epididymis.

estrogen A female hormone, produced by the developing egg follicles during the reproductive years, that causes stimulation of the uterine lining and changes in cervical mucus.

Fallopian tubes A pair of tubes that retrieve and carry the ova from the ovary to the uterus.

fertilization The union of egg and sperm.

fetus The developing embryo from the second month of gestation to birth.

fibroid tumors Benign uterine tumors composed of smooth muscle.

fimbriae The hairlike endings of the Fallopian tubes that retrieve the ovum as it is released from the ovary.

follicle-stimulating hormone (FSH) A hormone released by the pituitary gland that triggers ovum development or sperm production.

fost-adopt programs State or county programs that place children in foster homes as a first step in the adoption process.

fructose test A male fertility test that checks for the presence of fructose sugar in the semen.

FSH *See* follicle-stimulating hormone.

galactorrhea The presence of milk in the breasts of a woman who is not pregnant or has not recently given birth.

gamete intrafallopian tube transfer (GIFT) A procedure that removes one or more eggs from the female partner, mixes them with her mate's sperm, and then places them in the Fallopian tube for natural fertilization.

general anesthesia A type of anesthesia which induces unconsciousness.

genitals External sexual organs.

GIFT *See* gamete intrafallopian tube transfer.

gonadotropin-releasing hormone (GnRH) The hormone secreted by the hypothalamus that signals the pituitary to release FSH and LH hormones.

gonorrhea A bacterial, sexually transmitted disease.

Graafian follicle The dominant oocyte in the ovary, which will be ovulated.

gynecology A branch of medicine that specializes in the study and treatment of female reproduction, pregnancy, and birth.

gynecologist A doctor of medicine who specializes in female reproduction, pregnancy, and birth (also called an ob-gyn).

habitual aborter A medical term used to describe a woman who has miscarried three or more pregnancies.

hamster egg test Also called the sperm penetration assay; a male fertility test that checks the sperm's ability to penetrate a hamster ovum.

HCG *See* human chorionic gonadotropin.

heparin lock A device used to administer intravenous drugs.

HMG *See* human menopausal gonadotropin.

home study Part of the agency adoption qualifying process; a series of interviews and home visits with prospective adoptive parents.

hormones Secretions of the endocrine glands that trigger complex biochemical processes.

Huhner's test (or post-coital test/PCT) A workup test that assesses the quality and quantity of cervical mucus and how sperm react to it.

human chorionic gonadatropin (HCG) A hormone produced by the placenta during pregnancy; also used as a "fertility drug," in conjunction with HMG or clomiphene.

human menopausal gonadotropin (HMG) (Pergonal) A "fertility drug" composed of purified FSH and LH natural hormone, derived from the urine of postmenopausal women.

hyperprolactinism An excessive amount of prolactin hormone in the bloodstream.

hypothalamus The area of the brain near the pituitary gland that regulates hormonal secretions of the pituitary.

hyaluronidase An enzyme contained in the head of the sperm that aids in opening a path to the egg.

hysterectomy A surgical procedure that removes part or all of the uterus.

hysterosalpingogram (HSG) A work-up test that provides an X-ray picture of the uterus, tubes, and ovaries and checks tubal patency.

hysteroscopy Viewing the inside of the uterus through a narrow fitted telescope.

ICSH *See* interstitial cell stimulating hormone.

idiopathic oligospermia A low sperm count without known cause or pathology.

immunobead binding test A test to check for the presence and location of sperm antibodies on the sperm.

immobilization A condition in which the sperm are unable to move forward; they may be immobilized or "quiver and shake" in place.

immunological infertility Infertility caused by an immunologic reaction to sperm; may occur in either the male or female.

implantation The attachment of a fertilized egg to the uterine lining.

impotence The inability to achieve or maintain an erection.

incompetent cervix A weakened cervix that is unable to support the uterus as the fetus grows; may be the cause of second trimester miscarriages.

incomplete abortion A miscarriage in which not all the fetal tissue is expelled from the uterus.

independent or private adoption An increasingly popular type of adoption in which the birthparents and adoptive parents arrange the placement of the child themselves, usually with the assistance of a knowledgeable intermediary.

infertility The inability to conceive or maintain a pregnancy after one year of unprotected intercourse.

infertility specialist A gynecologist who has received further experience, education, and training to specialize in the diagnosis and treatment of infertility.

inflammation The reaction of the body's tissue to infection through swelling, pain, and/or scar formation.

infundibulum The trumpetlike end of the Fallopian tube, which nestles near the ovary.

inpatient surgery Usually "major" surgery for which the patient is hospitalized for several days or longer.

international adoption An adoption of a child from another country.

interstitial cell stimulating hormone (ICSH) The LH hormone in the male, which is instrumental in stimulating sperm production.

intrauterine device (IUD) A type of contraceptive, usually a "loop" or "shield," placed in the uterus; its use has been associated with salpingitis and infertility.

in vitro fertilization (IVF) An infertility treatment that extracts one or more eggs from the mother, fertilizes them with the father's sperm outside the body, and transfers the developing embryo(s) into the uterus to continue the pregnancy.

in vivo fertilization Fertilization occurring naturally within the body.

isthmus The narrow portion of a Fallopian tube, which is attached to the uterus.

IUD *See* intrauterine device.

IVF *See* in vitro fertilization.

karyotyping A test that photographs chromosomes for genetic information.

Klinefelter's syndrome A rare male disorder that involves an extra x chromosome.

laparoscopy A surgical procedure, often performed during the female infertility workup, in which the specialist views the reproductive organs through a special telescopelike instrument inserted near the navel.

laparotomy Opening of the abdomen by incision.

laser surgery A type of surgery that uses a laser beam either by itself or in conjunction with other microsurgical techniques.

Leydig cells Cells within the testes that manufacture testosterone.

LH *See* luteinizing hormone.

local anesthesia Injection of pain-numbing medicine directly into the skin or other tissues without inducing unconsciousness.

luteal phase The second half of the menstrual cycle—from ovulation to menses.

luteal phase defect A shortened luteal phase or one with inadequate progesterone production.

lutein A yellow pigment the body manufactures from cholesterol.

luteinizing hormone (LH) A pituitary hormone important to ovulation and progesterone production in women and testosterone production in men.

menarche The first menstrual period, usually occurring between the ages of 9 and 14.

menopause The last menstrual period after years of diminishing or erratic menses (the climacteric), commonly occurring between the ages of 45 and 55.

menstrual cycle The monthly cycle of ovulation, usually 25 to 35 days long.

menstruation The cyclical shedding of the endometrium when pregnancy does not occur.

microsurgery A delicate type of surgery performed through a microscope.

miscarriage The loss of a pregnancy, most often in the first trimester.

missed abortion A miscarriage where fetal tissue remains and symptoms have subsided.

motility The forward progression and movement of sperm.

natural childbirth Delivering a child vaginally without the use of anesthesia.

neonatal death The death of a newborn baby within a month of birth.

neonatalogist A pediatrician who has specialized training in the care of newborn (including premature) babies.

nidation Implantation of the fertilized ova into the uterus.

obstetrician A physician who specializes in female reproduction, pregnancy, and birth.

oligospermia A persistently subnormal sperm count.

oocyte An immature ovum.

open adoption A form of adoption in which some form of communication continues between the birthparents and the adoptive family.

orgasm In the male, sexual climax resulting in ejaculation; in the female, sexual climax usually through clitoral stimulation.

os Tiny opening of the cervix.

outpatient surgery Usually "minor" surgery performed in the hospital; patient is released the same day.

ovaries Female reproductive organs that store and release eggs during ovulation, as well as the hormones estrogen and progesterone.

oviduct The Fallopian tube.

ovulation The release of an ovum, or egg, from the ovary.

ovulation induction The stimulation of oocyte development and release through female hormone therapy.

ovulation pump A battery-run pump that administers gonadotropin-releasing hormone to induce ovulation.

ovum A female egg; plural, ova.

ovum transfer The transfer of a fertilized egg from a donor's to a recipient woman's uterus.

PAP smear test Analysis of a slide of cervical cells for abnormalities.

patration The action of the sperm opening a pathway to the ovum for those that follow.

pelvic inflammatory disease (PID) A catchall phrase referring to inflammation of the pelvis; most PID occurs in the Fallopian tubes.

penis The male sexual organ that excretes urine and ejaculates semen.

peristalsis Rhythmic contractions that move the sperm through the epididymis and vas deferens or move the egg through the Fallopian tube.

PID *See* pelvic inflammatory disease.

pipette A slender glass tube.

pituitary gland An endocrine gland, located near the base of the brain, that secretes various hormones and orchestrates the complex interactions of the menstrual cycle and spermatogenesis.

placenta previa A condition in which the placenta attaches between the fetus and the cervix.

polycystic ovarian syndrome A complex hormonal problem in which the ovaries fail to ovulate and instead form numerous tiny cysts.

post birth control pill syndrome The body's inability to resume ovulatory cycles following use of birth control pills.

pregnancy loss A miscarriage, ectopic pregnancy, or stillbirth.

premature ovarian failure A rare condition in which the ovary ceases functioning prematurely (before menopause should naturally occur.)

progesterone A female hormone produced by the ovaries in the second phase of the menstrual cycle.

prolactin A hormone secreted by the pituitary and associated with lactation.

proliferative phase The first half of the menstrual cycle, which culminates in ovulation.

prostaglandins Hormones that induce uterine contractions before menstruation or during labor.

prostate gland A male reproductive gland that contributes seminal fluids to the sperm before ejaculation.

RESOLVE A nationwide organization, founded in 1977 by Barbara Eck Menning, that provides referrals, support, and medical information to infertile individuals.

resolving infertility Confronting and grieving for the reality of infertility and then selecting the appropriate option (adoption, biological birth, child-free living).

retrograde bleeding The "backing-up" of menstrual fluid to the tubes, ovaries, or abdomen.

retrograde ejaculation A disorder of the male reproductive system in which semen is ejaculated into the bladder.

Rubin's test An outdated workup procedure that tests tubal patency by blowing carbon dioxide gas into the uterus.

salpingitis An infection of the Fallopian tubes, also called pelvic inflammatory disease (PID).

scrotum The saclike skin that covers the testicles.

secondary amenorrhea An absence of three or more consecutive menstrual cycles after puberty.

secondary infertility The inability to produce another child after one or more successful pregnancies.

secretory cells Fluid-secreting cells within the Fallopian tube.

secretory phase The second half of the menstrual cycle, which nourishes the fertilized egg or, if pregnancy does not occur, culminates in menstruation.

semen The thick (viscous), cloudy ejaculate that contains sperm and seminal fluids.

semen analysis A workup test that analyzes a sample of semen for sperm count, motility, morphology, and other characteristics.

seminal vesicles Small glands that store sperm and contribute much of the semen.

seminiferous tubules Tubes within the testes that produce sperm.

serum progesterone test A blood test, usually taken after ovulation, that measures the level of progesterone.

sexually transmitted disease (STD) Any of several dozen viral or bacterial diseases transmitted by genital, oral, or anal contact.

sperm The male germ cells, carrying genetic information, that fertilize an egg.

sperm antibodies Substances manufactured by men or women's immune systems that cause damage or destruction of sperm.

sperm bank A clinic that stores frozen donor sperm for use in artificial insemination.

sperm count A rough estimate of the number of sperm in a given "counting area."

sperm penetration assay Also called the hamster egg test; a male fertility test that checks the sperm's ability to penetrate a hamster ovum.

sperm washing A technique that separates the sperm from the seminal fluid.

spermatic cord The duct system that transports sperm from the testicle to the urethra for ejaculation.

spermatogenesis The process of sperm production.

spinal anesthesia An anesthetic injected into the spinal canal to produce numbness in a general area of the body, usually below the waist (for pelvic procedures or birthing).

Spinnbarkeit test A test that assesses the consistency and "stretchability" of cervical mucus.

split ejaculate Division of the semen into two samples; artificial insemination is usually tried with the first part, which contains most of the sperm.

spontaneous abortion Expelling of a fetus by the body during the first or second trimester; commonly termed miscarriage.

STD *See* sexually transmitted disease.

Stein-Leventhal syndrome *See* polycystic ovarian syndrome.

sterility Permanent, untreatable infertility.

stillbirth A third trimester fetus that has died in utero or during delivery.

superovulation The induction of several eggs through fertility drug treatment; usually used during in vitro fertilization.

surrogate mother A woman who contracts with a couple to bear the husband's biological child.

syphilis A sexually transmitted disease.

T-mycoplasma A microorganism that may be associated with infertility and miscarriage.

testes Male reproductive organs that produce sperm and male hormones.

testicular biopsy A procedure, performed under anesthesia, that removes a sample of tissue from the testicle.

testosterone A male hormone manufactured by the testes.

threatened abortion Vaginal staining and bleeding during pregnancy that may or may not result in a miscarriage.

thyroid The endocrine gland that secretes thyroxin hormone and helps maintain metabolism.

toxemia A pregnancy complication, usually occurring in the last trimester, that may include such symptoms as high blood pressure, swelling, and protein in the urine; requires immediate medical attention.

tubal patency An "open" tube without signs of blockage.

ultrasound A technique that bounces sound waves off the body to produce an image, often used to monitor ovarian activity or pregnancy.

unexplained infertility A "diagnosis" given to infertile couples for whom no organic problem can be detected in either partner.

urethra The tube that carries urine and semen through the penis.

urologist A physician who specializes in urinary tract diseases and male reproductive problems.

uterus The female reproductive organ that nurtures the fetus from implantation until birth.

vagina The muscular passage between the uterus and exterior vulva.

varicocele A varicose vein of the testicle.

vas deferens Two long ducts that connect the epididymis to the ejaculatory duct.

vasectomy A male sterilization procedure which severs the vas deferens.

vasectomy reversal A surgical procedure that repairs the severed vas deferens and hopefully restores fertility.

vasography An X-ray of the vas deferens.

vena cavae Two large veins that carry blood to the heart.

venereal disease A sexually transmitted disease; usually refers to syphilis or gonorrhea.

visualization A relaxation technique that employs calming, peaceful, and healing images.

zona pellucida The outer covering of the ovum that the sperm must penetrate before fertilization can occur.

zygote A fertilized ovum.

BIBLIOGRAPHY

General Infertility Readings

Barker, Graham H., M.D. *Your Search for Fertility: A Sympathetic Guide to Achieving Pregnancy for Childless Couples.* New York: Quill, 1983.

Bellina, Joseph H., M.D., Ph.D., and Josleen Wilson. *You CAN Have a Baby.* New York: Crown, 1985. A comprehensive guide to medical treatments now available for infertility.

Boston Women's Health Book Collective. "Infertility and Pregnancy Loss." Chapter 21 in *The New Our Bodies, Our Selves.* New York: Simon and Schuster, 1985.

Cooke, Cynthia, M.D., and Susan Dworkin. *The MS Guide to a Woman's Health.* New York: Anchor Books, 1979.

Corson, Stephen L., M.D. *Conquering Infertility.* Norwalk, Conn.: Appleton-Century-Crofts, 1983.

Decker, Albert, M.D., and Suzanne Lobel. *Why Can't We Have a Baby?* New York: Warner Books, 1978.

Fenton, Judith A., and Aaron S. Lifchez, M.D. *Fertility Handbook.* New York: Potter, 1980.

Harris, Diane, "What It Costs to Fight Infertility." *Money* 13 (December 1984): 201–212.

Harrison, Mary. *Infertility: A Couple's Guide to Its Causes and Treatments.* Boston: Houghton Mifflin, 1977.

Howard, James T., M.D., and Dodi Schultz. *We Want to Have a Baby.* New York: E. P. Dutton, 1979.

Jones, Howard W., M.D., and Georgeanna Seegar Jones, M.D. *Gynecology.* 3d ed. Baltimore: Williams & Wilkins, 1982.

Kaufman, Sherwin A., M.D. *You Can Have a Baby: New Hope for the Childless Couple.* New York: Bantam, 1978.

Madaras, Lynda, and Jane Patterson, M.D. *Womancare: A Gynecological Guide to Your Body.* New York: Avon, 1981.

Menning, Barbara Eck. *Infertility: A Guide for the Childless Couple.* Englewood Cliffs, N.J.: Prentice-Hall, 1977. The first comprehensive guide for infertility.

Nofziger, Margaret. *The Fertility Question.* New York: The Book Publishing Company, 1982.

Silber, Sherman J., M.D. *How to Get Pregnant.* New York: Warner, 1982.

Stangel, John H. *Fertility and Conception: An Essential Guide for the Childless Couple.* New York: North American Publishing, 1980.

Newsletters

Perspectives
Center for Communications in Infertility
P. O. Box 516
Yorktown Heights, NY 10598

RESOLVE, Inc.
5 Water Street
Arlington, MA 02174
(617) 643-2424
A quarterly newsletter issued by the national office. Various chapters around the country also publish periodic newsletters.

Stepping Stones
Central Christian Church in Wichita
P.O. Box 1141
Wichita, KS 67211

The Emotional Dynamics of Infertility

Anderson, Ann Kiemel. *Taste of Tears, Touch of God.* Nashville: Thomas Nelson Publications, 1984.

Berg, Barbara. *Nothing to Cry About.* New York: Seaview Books, 1981. Reissued by Bantam, 1983.

Bombardieri, Merle. "The Twenty Minute Rule: First Aid for Couples in Distress." *RESOLVE National Newsletter* (December 1983), 5.

Bunker, John, *et al. Costs, Risks, and Benefits of Surgery.* New York: Oxford University Press, 1977.

Burns, Cheri. *Stepmotherhood.* New York: Time Books, 1985.

Chiappone, Janice M. "Infertility as a Nonevent: Impact, Coping, and Differences Between Men and Women." Ph.D. Diss., University of Maryland, 1984.

Fleming, Jeanne, Ph.D. "Infertility as a Chronic Illness." *RESOLVE National Newsletter* (December 1984).

Fleming, Jeanne, Ph.D., and Kenneth A. Burry, M.D., "Coping with Infertility: How Infertile People Process Grief." Paper presented to the National Annual Convention of the American Fertility Society, Chicago, October 1985.

Halvorsen, Kaye, and Karen Hess. *The Wedded Unmother.* Minneapolis: Augsburg Publishing, 1980.

Hanes, Mari, and Jack Hayford. *Beyond Heartache.* Wheaton, Ill.: Tyndale House, 1984.

Huneycutt, Harry C., M.D., and Judith L. Davis. *All About Hysterectomy.* New York: Reader's Digest Press, 1977.

Johnston, Patricia Irwin. *Understanding: A Guide to Impaired Fertility for Family and Friends.* Fort Wayne, Ind.: Perspectives Press, 1983.

McGowan, Joan Y. Waiting: *The Hope and Frustrations of a Childless Couple.* New York: Vantage Press, 1983.

Menning, Barbara Eck, R.N., "The Emotional Needs of Infertile Couples." *Fertility and Sterility* 34, no. 4 (1980): 313–319.

Mitchard, Jacquelyn. *Mother Less Child.* New York: W. W. Norton, 1985.

Morgan, Susanne. *Coping with a Hysterectomy.* New York: Dial Press, 1983.

Salzer, Linda P. *Infertility: How Couples Can Cope.* Boston: G. K. Hall, 1986.

Stigger, Judith A. *Coping with Infertility.* Minneapolis: Augsburg Publishing, 1983.

Stout, Martha. *Without Child: A Compassionate Look at Infertility.* Grand Rapids, Mich.: Zondervan, 1985.

Taking Care of Yourself

Bailey, Covert. *Fit or Fat?* Boston: Houghton Mifflin, 1978.

Boston Women's Health Book Collective. *Our Bodies, Our Selves* and *The New Our Bodies, Our Selves.* New York: Simon & Schuster, 1976 and 1985.

Brown, Barbara. *Stress and the Art of Biofeedback.* New York: Harper & Row, 1977.

Charlesworth, Edward A., Ph.D., and Ronald G. Nathan, Ph.D. *Stress Management.* New York: Ballantine, 1984.

Cooper, Mildred, and Kenneth H. Cooper, M.D. *Aerobics for Women.* New York: Bantam, 1972.

Cousins, Norman. *Anatomy of an Illness.* New York: W. W. Norton, 1979.

Duff, William. *Sugar Blues.* Radnor, Pa.: Chilton Book Co., 1975.

Fonda, Jane. *Workout Book.* New York: Simon & Schuster, 1981.

Lappe, Frances Moore. *Diet for a Small Planet.* New York: Ballantine Books, 1975.

Mason, L. John, Ph.D. *Guide to Stress Reduction.* Culver City, Calif.: Peace Press, 1980.

Nierenberg, Judith, R.N., and Florence Janovic. *The Hospital Experience: A Guide for Patients and Their Families.* New York: Berkley Publishing, 1985.

Notman, Malkah T., M.D., and Carol Nadelson, M.D., eds. *The Woman Patient: Medical and Psychological Interfaces.* New York: Plenum Publishing, 1982.

Robertson, Laurel, Carol Flinders and Brian Ruttenhal. *Laurel's Kitchen.* Berkeley, Calif.: Ten Speed Press, 1986.

Samuels, Mike, M.D., and Nancy Samuels. *Seeing with the Mind's Eye.* New York: Random House, 1975.

_____. *The Well Body Book.* New York: Random House, 1976.

Sheehy, Gail. *Passages.* New York: Bantam Books, 1976.

Simonton, Carl, M.D., and Stephanie Matthews Simonton. *Getting Well Again.* New York: Bantam, 1980.

Weiss, Kay, M.P.H., ed. *Women's Health Care: A Guide to Alternatives.* Reston, Va.: Reston Publishing, 1984.

Hormonal Problems and Their Treatment

Evrard, J.R., et al. "Amenorrhea Following Oral Contraceptives." *American Journal of Obstetrics and Gynecology* 124 (1976) 88–91.

"Fertility Boost: Hormones Plus Pump." *Science News* 124 (July 1983) 59.

Goldzicher, J. W. "Polycystic Ovarian Disease." *Fertility and Sterility* 35, no. 4 (April 1981) 371–394.

Graedon, Joe, and Teresa Graedon. *The New People's Pharmacy: Drug Breakthroughs of the '80s.* New York: Bantam, 1985.

Meyers, Robert. *The Bitter Pill.* New York: Seaview Books, 1983.

Paul, Michele, R.N. *The Women's Pharmacy: What Every Woman Should Know about the Medicines for Her Feminine Problems.* New York: Simon & Schuster, 1983.

Rayburn, William F., M.D., Frederick Zuspun, M.D., and Jeanne Fitzgerald. *Every Woman's Pharmacy.* New York: Doubleday, 1984.

RESOLVE, Inc. "Luteal Phase Defect." 1980. Fact sheet available from the national office and many local chapters.

"The PMS Connection," Newsletter about PMS, P.O. Box 9326, Madison, WI 53715.

Pelvic Abnormalities and Microsurgery Treatment

Bichler, Joyce. *DES Daughter.* New York: Avon Books, 1981.

Englemayer, Sheldon, and Robert Wagman. *Lord's Justice.* New York: Doubleday, 1986. The legal investigation and hearings on the Dalkon Shield.

Fertility and Pregnancy Guide for DES Daughters and Sons. DES Action, USA, West Coast Office, 2845–24th St., San Francisco, CA 94110, (415) 621-8032. Extensive presentation of the medical literature and interviews with DES specialists.

Herbst, Arthur L. "Reproductive and Gynecologic Surgical Experience in DES-exposed Daughters." *American Journal of Obstetrics and Gynecology* 14, no. 8 (December 1981): 1019-1028.

Jacobson, Lennart, M.D. "Differential Diagnosis of Acute Pelvic Inflammatory Disease." *American Journal of Obstetrics and Gynecology* 138, no. 7, pt. 2 (December 1, 1980): 1006–1011.

Kaufman, D. W., et al. "Intrauterine Contraceptive Device Use and Pelvic Inflammatory Disease." *American Journal of Obstetrics and Gynecology* 136 (1980): 159–62.

Mintz, Morton. *At Any Cost.* New York: Pantheon, 1986. Discussion of the ethics of using the Dalkon Shield.

"More Bad News About Sex." *Newsweek,* April 21, 1986, 70–71. Update on the sexually transmitted disease, chlamydia.

Orenberg, Cynthia L., and Robert Meyers. *DES: The Complete Story.* New York: St. Martin's Press, 1981.

Roberts, Katherine. "The Intrauterine Device as a Health Risk." *Women and Health,* July/August 1977, 21–30.

Vancouver Women's Health Research Collective. *P.I.D.: Pelvic Inflammatory Disease.* Vancouver: 1983. An excellent illustrated booklet, which also contains a bibliography. At this printing, available for $2 from VWHRC, 1501 W. Broadway, Vancouver, B.C., Canada V6J 1W6.

Endometriosis

Dmowski, W. P. "Current Concepts in the Management of Endometriosis." *Obstetrics and Gynecology Annual* 10 (1981): 279–311.

Older, Julia A. *A Woman's Guide to Endometriosis.* New York: Charles Scribner's Sons, 1984. A comprehensive discussion of the causes, treatments, and myths about endometriosis. Cites many other articles and books about the subject.

Immunological and Unexplained Infertility

Bronson, Richard, M.D., George Cooper, Ph.D., and David Rosenfeld, M.D. "Sperm Antibodies: Their Role in Infertility." *Fertility and Sterility* 42, no. 2 (1984): 171–183.

Morse, G. "Sperm Antibodies Frustrate Fertility." *Science News* 126 (July 1984): 38.

Mumford, David M., M.D., "Immunology and Male Infertility." *Urologic Clinics of North America* 5, no. 3 (1978): 463–480.

Shulman, Sidney, et al. "New Method of Treatment of Immunological Infertility." *Urology* (November 1978): 582–586.

"When You Suspect Infertility Is Immunologic." *Contemporary OB/GYN* 14 (November 1979): 92–113.

Pregnancy Loss: Medical Facts and Emotional Aftermath

Borg, Susan, and Judith Lasker. *When Pregnancy Fails: Families Coping with Miscarriage, Stillbirth, and Infant Death.* Boston: Beacon Press, 1981.

Boston Women's Health Collective. *The New Our Bodies, Our Selves.* New York: Simon & Schuster, 1985.

Doelp, Alan. *Autumn's Children: A Real Life Drama of High Risk Pregnancy.* New York: Macmillan, 1985.

Elliman, Wendy. "Making a Carriage from Miscarriage." *Hadassah* 66, no. 9 (May 1985): 40–43. Discussion of the treatment of acquired antibody, "Lupus antiocagulant," which may cause repeated pregnancy loss.

Friedman, Rochelle, M.D., and Bonnie Gradstein, M.P.H. *Surviving Pregnancy Loss.* Boston: Little, Brown, 1982.

Grollman, Earl A. *Explaining Death to Children.* Boston: Beacon Press, 1967.

Kübler-Ross, Elisabeth. *On Children and Dying.* New York: Collier, 1983.

_____. *On Death and Dying.* New York: Macmillan, 1970.

Panuthos, Claudia. *Ended Beginnings: Healing Childbearing Losses.* South Hadley, Mass.: Bergin & Garvey, 1984.

Pepper, Larry G., Ph.D., and Ronald J. Knapp, Ph.D. *How to Go on Living After the Death of a Baby.* Atlanta: Peachtree Publishers, 1985.

Seiden, Othnel J., M.D., and M. J. Timmons, R.N. *Coping with Miscarriage.* Blue Ridge Summit, Pa.: TAB Books, 1984.

New Frontiers: IVF, Gift, and Embryo Transfers

Adamson, David, M.D. "Gamete Intra-Fallopian Transfer." *RESOLVE Northern California Chapter Newsletter* 7, no. 3 (October 1985): 6–7.

American Fertilization Society. "Ethical Statement on In Vitro Fertilization." *Fertility and Sterility* 41, no. 12 (1984).

American Fertility Society. "Minimal Standards for Programs of In Vitro Fertilization." *Fertility and Sterility* 41, no. 13 (1984).

Andrews, Lori B., J.D. *New Conceptions.* New York: Ballantine, 1985.

_____. "Yours, Mine and Theirs." *Psychology Today.* 18, no. 20 (December 1984): 20–29.

Arditti, Rita, Renate Duelli Klein, and Shelley Minden. *Test-Tube Women: What Future for Motherhood?* Boston: Routledge & Kegan Paul, 1984. Raises questions about how in vitro fertilization is performed and how women and men are treated in high-tech medical procedures.

Brotman, H. "Human Embryo Transplants." *New York Times Magazine,* 8 January 1984.

Clapp, Diane, R.N., B.S.N., and Merle Bombardieri, L.C.S.W. "Easing Stress for IVF Patients and Staff." *Contemporary OB/GYN* 24; no. 4 (October 1984): 91–99.

Corea, Genoveffa. *The Mother Machine: Reproductive Technologies from Artificial Insemination to Artificial Wombs.* New York: Harper & Row, 1985. A look at the high-tech birth options being developed and the ethical issues they raise.

"Ending Infertility with Ovum Transfers." *Newsweek,* 1 August 1983, 48.

Glass, Robert H., M.D., and Ronald Ericcson, Ph.D. *Getting Pregnant in the 1980's: New Advances in Infertility Treatment and Sex Pre-Selection.* Berkeley: University of California Press, 1982.

Gold, Michael. "Franchising Test Tube Babies." *Science,* April 1986, 16–17.

"The New Origins of Life." *Time,* 10 September 1984, 46–53.

Olson, Maleia, R.N., and Nancy J. Alexander, Ph.D. *In Vitro Fertilization and Embryo Transfer.* Portland, Ore.: The Oregon Health Sciences University, 1984. Excellent pamphlet about IVF. Write for current cost and ordering information: In Vitro Program, Oregon Health Sciences University, 3181 S. W. Sam Jackson Park Road, Portland, OR 97201.

Singer, Peter, and Deane Wells. *Making Babies: The New Science and Ethics of Conception.* New York: Charles Scribner's Sons, 1985. A thorough look at the techniques and ethics of IVF and other high-tech infertility treatments; contains a comprehensive bibliography.

Tilton, Nan, Todd Tilton, and Gaylen Moore. *Making Miracles: In Vitro Fertilization.* Garden City, N.Y.: Doubleday, 1985.

Wood, Carl and Ann Westmore. *Test Tube Conceptions.* New York: Prentice-Hall, 1984.

Male Infertility and Artificial Insemination

Alexander, Nancy J., Ph.D., John H. Sampson, M.D., and Miles J. Nory, M.D. *Artificial Insemination.* Portland, Ore.: Oregon Health Sciences University, 1981.

Amelar, Richard, M.D., Laurence Dubin, M.D., and Patricia Walsh, M.D. *Male Infertility.* Philadelphia: W. B. Saunders, 1977.

Binor, Z., J. E. Sokoloski, and D. P. Wold. "Penetration of the Zona Free Hamster Egg by Human Sperm." *Fertility and Sterility* 33 (1980): 321.

Carlson, J. "Swimmingly Successful Sperm." *Health* 15 (November 1983): 14.

Cohen-Curie, Martin, Lesleigh Luttrell, and Sander Shapiro. "Current Practice of Artificial Insemination by Donor in the United States." *New England Journal of Medicine* 300, no. 11 (15 March 1984): 585–90.

Greenberg, S. H. "Varicocele and Male Infertility." *Fertility and Sterility* 28 (1977): 699.

Lipschultz, Larry L., M.D., and Stuart S. Howard, M.D. *Infertility in the Male.* New York: Churchill-Livingstone, 1983.

Mascola, Laurene, M.D., and Mary E. Guinan, M.D. "Screening to Reduce Transmission of Sexually Transmitted Diseases in Semen Used for Artificial Insemination." *The New England Journal of Medicine* 314 (1986): 1354–1359.

McClure, R. Dale, M.D. "The Zona Free Hamster Egg Penetration Test: Its Usefulness in Male Infertility." *Seminars in Urology* 3, no. 2 (May 1985) 78–84.

Overstreet, James, M.D., R. Yanagimachi, M.D., and D. F. Katz, M.D., et al. "Penetration of Human Spermatozoa into the Human Zona Pellucida and the Zona Free Hamster Egg: A Study of Fertile Donors and Infertile Patients." *Fertility and Sterility* 33 (1980): 534–542.

Sharlip, Ira D., M.D. "Clinical Andrology." In *General Urology,* 11th ed. Palo Alto, Calif. : Lange Medical Series, 1984.

Silber, Sherman J., M.D. *How to Get Pregnant.* New York: Charles Scribner's Sons, 1980. An excellent reference book, particularly informative about male psychology and infertility.

_____. *The Male: From Infancy to Old Age.* New York: Charles Scribner's Sons, 1981.

Walzer, H., M.D. "Psychological and Legal Aspects of Artificial Insemination: An Overview." *American Journal of Psychotherapy* 36 (1982): 91–103.

Adoption

General Readings

American Council on Adoptable Children. *Adoption Booklet.* A free guide on state departments of social services, adoptive parent groups, and transracial and intercountry adoptions. Write to NACAC, 1346 Connecticut Ave., N.W., Suite 229, Washington, D.C. 20036.

Arms, Suzanne. *To Love and Let Go.* New York: Alfred A. Knopf, 1983. A poignant look at the stories of several birthmothers and adoptive parents, with an advocacy for an open approach to adoption.

Benet, Mary K. *The Politics of Adoption.* New York: Free Press, 1976. An experienced social worker's perspective.

Berman, Claire. *We Take This Child: A Candid Look at Modern Adoption.* Garden City, N.Y.: Doubleday, 1974.

Bolles, Edmund Blair. *The Penguin Adoption Book.* New York: Penguin, 1984.

Burgess, Linda Cannon. *The Art of Adoption*. Washington, D.C.: Acropolis Books, 1978. A progressive social worker reflects on her adoption placement experiences and triad member issues.

Canape, Charlene. *Adoption: Parenthood Without Pregnancy.* New York: Henry Holt, 1986. The author's personal experience with adoption; contains excellent appendices of adoption agencies and support groups across the country.

Dywarsuk, Collette T. *Adoption: Is It For You?* New York: Harper & Row, 1973. A good handbook for couples interested in adoption.

Gilman, Lois. "Adoption: How to Do It on Your Own." *Money* 14, no. 10 (October, 1985) 161–168.

_____. *The Adoption Resource Book*. New York: Harper & Row, 1984.

Gradstein, Bonnie, M.P.H., Marc Gradstein, J.D., and Robert H. Glass, M.D. "Private Adoption." *Fertility and Sterility.* 37, no. 4 (April 1982): 548–552.

Kirk, H. David. *Shared Fate*. New York: Free Press, 1964.

Leavy, Norton L. *Laws of Adoption*. Dobbs Ferry, N.Y.: Ocean Press, 1968. Contains adoption laws in each state, which may be somewhat outdated.

Martin, Cynthia. *Beating the Adoption Game.* La Jolla, Calif.: Oaktree Publications, 1980.

McNamara, Joan. *The Adoption Adviser.* New York: Hawthorn Books, 1975.

McWhinnie, A. M. *Adopted Children and How They Grow Up*. London: Routledge & Kegan Paul, 1967.

Munzan, William, Sanford Katz, and Eva Russo. *Adoptions without Agencies: A Study of Independent Adoptions*. New York: CWLA, 1978.

Paton, Jean M. *Orphan Voyage*. New York: Vantage, 1978.

Plumez, Jacqueline Hornor. *Successful Adoption: A Guide to Finding a Child and Raising a Family.* New York: Harmony Books, 1982. Good general reference book.

Public Affairs Pamphlets: *So You Want to Adopt a Baby, #173,* and *You and Your Adopted Child, #274*. Can be ordered from 381 Park Avenue South, New York, NY 10016. Write them for current prices.

Powledge, Fred. *The New Adoption Maze and How to Get Through It*. St. Louis, Mo.: C. V. Mosby, 1985.

Raymond, Louise. *Adoption and After.* New York: Harper & Row, 1974. An examination of adoption and its lifelong issues.

Rillera, Mary Jo, and Sharon Kaplan. *Cooperative Adoption: A Handbook*. Westminster, Calif.: Triadoption Publications, 1984.

Roberts, January, and Diane C. Robie. *Open Adoption and Open Placement*. Brooklyn Park, Minn.: Adoption Press, 1981.

Rondell, Florence, and Ruth Michaels. *The Adopted Family.* 2 vols. New York: Crown, 1965. A reference for the entire family. Volume 1, *The Adopted Family,* discusses the differences between biological and adopted families. Volume 2,

The Family That Grew, is devoted to a loving, sensitive understanding of the adopted child. Appropriate from age 5 and up.

Smith, Jerome, Ph.D., and Franklin Miroff, J.D. *You're Our Child: A Social/Psychological Approach to Adoption.* Washington, D.C.: University Press of America, 1981.

Warren, Jeanne Lindsay. *Open Adoption: A Caring Option.* Buena Park, Calif.: Morning Glory Press, 1987. Advocacy for open adoption, especially sensitive to the birthmother's position.

Wishard, Laura, and William R. Wishard. *The Grafted Tree.* San Francisco: Cragmont Publications, 1979.

Children's Books About Adoption

Beatty, P. *That's One Ornery Orphan.* New York: William Morrow, 1980.

Bunin, C., and S. Bunin. *Is That Your Sister?* New York: Pantheon Books, 1976. Appropriate for young children, a photo story written by a mother and daughter.

Caines, J. *Abby.* New York: Harper & Row, 1973.

Chinnock, F. *Kim: A Gift from Vietnam.* New York: World Publishers, 1969. The story of Kim's international adoption from the start through her first year in the United States.

Gordon, S. *The Boy Who Wanted a Family.* New York: Harper & Row, 1980. For ages 6 and older, a story about a 7-year-old foster child adopted by a single mother.

Krementz, Jill. *How It Feels to Be Adopted.* New York: Alfred A. Knopf, 1982. Photos and essays in adopted children's own words.

Lapsley, S. *I Am Adopted.* New York: Bodley Head, 1984. For young children.

Lifton, Betty J. *I'm Still Me.* New York: Alfred A. Knopf, 1981. Fiction story about an adolescent girl's search. Ages 14 and older.

Livingston, Carole. *Why Was I Adopted?* Secaucus, N.J.: Lyle Stuart, 1978. Excellent child's book about adoption.

Powledge, Fred. *So You're Adopted.* New York: Charles Scribner's Sons, 1982. A discussion of the different feelings adoptees have. For ages 14 and older.

Purcell, M. *A Look at Adoption.* New York: Lerner, 1978. For young children, a lovely book with photographs.

Silman, R. *Somebody Else's Child.* New York: F. Warne, 1976. Novel about adoption for ages 8 and older.

Stein, A. Bonnett. *The Adopted One.* New York: Walker, 1979. A book for kids and parents, with photographs.

Wasson, V. P. *The Chosen Baby.* New York: J. B. Lippincott, 1939. A young child's book about agency adoption.

Waybill, M. *Chinese Eyes.* New York: Herald Press, 1974. For ages 6 and older, a discussion about being different.

International Adoption

American Public Welfare Association. *Intercountry Adoption Guidelines.* Washington, D.C.: U. S. Government Printing Office, 1980.

_____. *National Directory of Intercountry Adoption Services Resources.* Washington, D.C.: U. S. Government Printing Office, 1980.

deHartog, Jan. *The Children.* New York: Atheneum, 1969. The adoptive family's reactions and adjustments to the adoption of two Korean girls.

Holt, B. *Seed from the East, Outstretched Arms.* London: Oxford Press, 1956, 1972. The story of the Holt Agency, which facilitates international adoptions.

Nelson-Erichsen, Jean, and Heino R. Erichsen. *Gamines: How to Adopt from Latin America.* Minneapolis: Dillon Press, 1981.

Viguers, Susan T. *With Child: One Couple's Journey to Their Adopted Children.* San Diego: Harcourt Brace Jovanovich, 1986.

Special Needs Adoption

Blank, P. *Nineteen Steps Up the Mountain: The Story of the DeBolt Family.* Philadelphia: J. B. Lippincott, 1976. The story of a remarkable family that has adopted many kids from various racial, international, and special needs backgrounds.

Carney, Ann. *No More Here and There: Adopting the Older Child.* North Carolina: University of North Carolina Press, 1976.

Jewett, Claudia L. *Adopting the Older Child.* Harvard, Mass.: Harvard Common Press, 1978. Coping with the unique needs of older children.

McNamara, J., and B. McNamara. *The Special Child Handbook.* New York: Hawthorn Books, 1977.

Rondell, Florence, and Ann Murray. *New Dimensions in Adoption.* New York: Crown Publishers, 1974. A handbook for adoption of special needs children and those from other countries.

Transracial Adoption

Anderson, David C. *Children of Special Value: Interracial Adoption in America.* New York: St. Martin's Press, 1971.

Ladner, Joyce. *Mixed Families: Adopting across Racial Boundaries.* New York: Anchor Books, 1978. Excellent discussion of transracial adoption and its challenges.

Lund, T. *Patchwork Clan: How the Sweeney Clan Grew.* New York: Little, Brown, 1932. Story of a large transracial family, their challenges and triumphs.

Simon, Rita J., and Howard Alstein. *Transracial Adoption.* New York: John Wiley, 1977.

Triad Member Issues

Askin, I. Jayne, and Bob Oskam. *Search: A Handbook for Adoptees and Birthparents.* New York: Harper & Row, 1982.

Brown, Dirck, et al. *Dialogue for Understanding: A Handbook for Adoptive and Pre-Adoptive Parents,* 2 vols. Palo Alto, Calif.: PACER, 1981. Perspectives from all triad members. Available from Post Adoption Center for Education and Research, 2255 Ygnacio Valley Rd., Suite L, Walnut Creek, CA 94598.

Campbell, Lee. *Understanding the Birth Parent.* Milford, Mass.: Concerned United Birthparents, 1978.

Cheetham, Juliet. *Unwanted Pregnancy and Counseling.* London: Routledge & Kegan Paul, 1977.

DuPrau, Jeanne. *Adoption: The Facts, Feelings and Issues of a Double Heritage.* New York: Simon & Schuster, 1981. A comprehensive discussion of the issues for all triad members.

Dusky, Lorraine. *Birthmark.* New York: Evans, 1974. A birthmother describes her feelings about relinquishing her daughter.

Ehrlich, Henry. *A Time to Search.* New York: Paddington Press, 1978. Account of a dozen searches and reunions.

Fisher, Florence. *The Search for Anna Fisher.* New York: Arthur Fields, 1973. The founder of Adoptees Liberty Movement Association (ALMA) describes her search for her birthparents.

Hulse, Jerry, and Helen Jo Hulse. *Jody.* New York: McGraw-Hill, 1976. An adoptee's search.

Johnston, Patricia Irwin, ed. *Perspectives on a Grafted Tree.* Fort Wayne, Ind.: Perspectives Press, 1983. A collection of poetry by and about those touched by adoption.

Lifton, Betty J. *Lost and Found: The Adoption Experience.* New York: Dial Press, 1983. The author's poignant and somewhat bitter look at her adoption experience.

_____. *Twice Born: Memories of an Adopted Daughter.* New York: McGraw-Hill, 1977. Author's story of her search for her birthparents.

Lindsay, Jeanne Warren. *Pregnant Too Soon: Adoption Is an Option.* Buena Park, Calif.: Morning Glory Press, 1980.

Rillera, Mary Jo. *The Adoption Searchbook: Techniques for Tracing People.* Huntington Beach, Calif.: Tri-Adoption Publishers, 1981.

Silber, Kathleen, and P. Speelin. *Dear Birthmother.* San Antonio, Tex.: Adoption Awareness Press, 1982.

Sorosky, Arthur D., M.D., Annette Baron, M.S.W., and Reuben Pannor, M.S.W. *The Adoption Triangle: The Effects of the Sealed Record on Adoptees, Birth Parents, and Adoptive Parents.* New York: Anchor Press, 1978. An advocacy for reform of the present adoption system.

Biological Birth

Arms, Suzanne. *Immaculate Deception*. New York: Houghton-Mifflin, 1974.

Bing, Elisabeth, and Libby Colman. *Having a Baby After 30*. New York: Bantam, 1980.

_____. *Making Love During Pregnancy*. New York: Bantam, 1974.

Boston Women's Health Book Collective. *Ourselves and Our Children*. New York: Random House, 1978.

Donovan, Bonnie. *The Cesarian Birth Experience*. Boston: Beacon Press, 1977.

Elkins, Valmai H. *The Rights of the Pregnant Parent*. New York: Schocken Books, 1976.

Fay, Francesca C., and Kathy Smith. *Childbearing after 35: The Risks and Rewards*. New York: Balsam Press, 1985.

Goldberg, Larry H., M.D. and Joann Leahy, M.D. *The Doctor's Guide to Medication During Pregnancy and Lactation*. New York: Quill, 1984.

Hotchner, Tracy. *Pregnancy and Childbirth*. New York: Avon, 1984.

Karmel, Marjorie. *Painless Childbirth—Thank You, Dr. Lamaze*. New York: Dolphin, 1965.

Milinaire, Caterine. *Birth*. New York: Harmony Books, 1971.

Nilsson, Lennart. *A Child Is Born*. New York: Delta, 1966.

Price, Jane. *You're Not Too Old to Have a Baby*. New York: Farrar, Straus & Giroux, 1977.

Pryor, Karen. *Nursing Your Baby*. New York: Pocket Books, 1973.

Weaver, Nell. *Your Fit Pregnancy*. Mountain View, Calif.: Anderson World Books, 1984.

Surrogate Mothers

"Infertility: Babies by Contract." *Newsweek*, 4 November 1985, 74–77.

Keane, Noel P. and Dennis Breo. *The Surrogate Mother*. New York: Everest House, 1981.

Menning, Barbara Eck. "Surrogate Motherhood: What Are the Ethical Issues?" *RESOLVE National Newsletter*, June 1981, 6–7.

"Surrogate Mothers: For Whom Are They Working?" *MS.*, March 1983, 18–20.

"Surrogate Mothers: The Legal Issues," *American Journal of Law and Medicine* 7, no. 3 (Fall 1981) 323–352.

vanHoften, Ellen Lassner. "Surrogate Mothers in California: Legislative Proposals." *San Diego Law Review* 18; no. 2 (March 1981): 341–385.

Parenting

Brazleton, T. Berry, M.D. *Infants and Mothers.* New York: Delta, 1970.

Caplan, Frank. *The First Twelve Months of Life.* New York: Bantam, 1978.

Church, Joseph. *Understanding Your Child from Birth to Three.* New York: Random House, 1973.

Gesell, Arnold, M.D. *The First Five Years of Life.* New York: Harper & Row, 1940.

Ginott, Hiam G. *Between Parent and Child.* New York: Avon, 1969.

Halaby, Mona, and Helen Neville, R.N. *No Fault Parenting.* New York: Facts on File, 1985.

Ilg, Frances L., M.D. and Louise Bates Ames, Ph.D. *Child Behavior: From Birth to Ten.* New York: Harper & Row, 1955.

Jewett, Claudia. *Helping Children Cope with Separation and Loss.* Boston: Harvard Press, 1982. Guidance for helping kids cope with past and present losses such as relinquishment, divorce, and death.

Kelly, Marguerite, and Elia Parsons. *The Mother's Almanac.* New York: Doubleday, 1975. Excellent book for new parents about the realities of childrearing.

Klein, Carole. *The Single Parent Experience.* New York: Avon, 1973.

Merritt, Sharyne, and Linda Steiner. *And Baby Makes Two: Motherhood without Marriage.* New York: Franklin Watts, 1984.

Pogrebin, Letty Cottin. *Growing Up Free: Raising Your Child in the 80's.* New York: McGraw-Hill, 1980.

Spock, Benjamin, M.D. *Baby and Child Care.* New York: Hawthorn Books, 1976.

Child-Free Living

Bombardieri, Merle. *The Baby Decision: How to Make the Most Important Choice of Your Life.* New York: Rawson, Wade Publishers, 1981.

_____. "Child-free Decision-Making," a 12-page reprint discussing the issues of child-free living, available from RESOLVE's national office.

Burgwyn, Diana. *Marriage Without Children.* New York: Harper & Row, 1981.

Covington, Sharon, L.C.S.W. "Child-free: The 'Closet Choice'" *RESOLVE, Washington, D.C. Metropolitan Chapter Newsletter,* May 1985.

Fabe, Marilyn, and Norma Wikler. *Up Against the Clock: Career Women Speak on the Choice to Have Children.* New York: Random House, 1979.

Faux, Marian. *Childless by Choice: Choosing Childlessness in the Eighties.* New York: Doubleday, 1984.

Feldman, Silvia. *Making Up Your Mind about Motherhood.* New York: Bantam, 1985.

Peck, Ellen. *The Baby Trap.* New York: Bernard Geis Associates, 1971.

Peck, Ellen, and Judy Senderowitz, eds. *Pronatalism: The Myth of Mom and Apple Pie.* New York: T. Y. Crowell, 1974.

Poole, William E. "Fathering Without Children." *San Francisco Examiner Image Magazine,* 3 November 1985.

Silverman, Anna, and Arnold Silverman. *The Case Against Having Children.* New York: David McKay, 1971.

Sullivan, Judy. *Mama Doesn't Live Here Anymore.* New York: Arthur Field Books, 1974.

Whelan, Elizabeth. *A Baby? Maybe.* New York: Bobbs-Merrill, 1975.

APPENDIX A

Resources

Medical Information, Referrals, and Emotional Support

AMERICAN ASSOCIATION OF GYNECOLOGIC LAPAROSCOPISTS
11239 S. Lakewood Blvd.
Downey, CA 90241

AMERICAN FERTILITY SOCIETY
1608 13th Ave. S., Suite 101
Birmingham, AL 35256

THE COMPASSIONATE FRIENDS
PO Box 1347
Oak Brook, IL 60521
(312) 323-5010
(A nationwide organization for parents who have lost a child)

DES ACTION, USA
National Offiice
Long Island Jewish Medical Center
New Hyde Park, NY 11040
(516) 775-3450

DES ACTION, USA
West Coast Office
2845 24th St.
San Francisco, CA 94110
(415) 826-5060

THE ENDOMETRIOSIS ASSOCIATION
PO Box 92187
Milwaukee, WI 53202
(414) 962-9031

GYNECOLOGIC LASER SOCIETY
500 Blue Hills Ave.
Hartford, CT 06112

THE PLANETREE HEALTH RESOURCE CENTER
2040 Webster St.
San Francisco, CA 94115
(415) 923-3680
(Library, bookstore, and medical information research service)

RESOLVE, INC.
National Office
5 Water St.
Arlington, MA 02174
(617) 643-2424
(The National Office has referrals for specialists and medical information and can also direct you to a local chapter near your home.)

Adoption Resources

AASK AMERICA
(Aid to Adoption of Special Kids)
3530 Grand Ave.
Oakland, CA 94610
(415) 451-1748

ADOPTED CHILD
PO Box 9362
Moscow, ID 83843
(Monthly newsletter to assist parents with daily realities of adoption. For subscription information, call 1(800) 635-8574.)

ADOPTEES BIRTHRIGHTS COMMITTEE
PO Box 3932
Lafayette, LA 70502

ADOPTEES IN SEARCH
PO Box 41016
Bethesda, MD 20014

ADOPTEES LIBERTY MOVEMENT ASSOCIATION (ALMA)
PO Box 154
Washington Bridge Station
New York, NY 10033

ADOPTION SERVICES OF WACAP
PO Box 2009
Port Angeles, WA 98362

MARTIN BRANDFON
Independent Search Consultant
PO Box 1923
Burlingame, CA 94010

CHILD WELFARE LEAGUE OF AMERICA (CWLA)
67 Irving Place
New York, NY 10003

COMMITTEE FOR SINGLE ADOPTIVE PARENTS
PO Box 4074
Chevy Chase, MD 20815

CONCERNED UNITED BIRTHPARENTS (CUB)
595 Central Ave.
Dover, NH 03820

FAMILIES ADOPTING INTER-RACIALLY (F.A.I.R)
989 Woodland
Menlo Park, CA 94025

INTERNATIONAL SOUNDEX REUNION REGISTRY
PO Box 2312
Carson City, NV 89701

NATIONAL ADOPTION RESOURCE EXCHANGE (NARE)
67 Irving Place
New York, NY
(212) 254-7410
(Devoted to finding homes for kids with special needs and minority children)

NATIONAL COMMITTEE FOR ADOPTION
1346 Connecticut Ave. NW, Suite 326
Washington, DC 20036
(202) 463-7559
(Promotes adoption as a positive family building option. Hotline provides information and referrals: (202) 463-7563.)

NORTH AMERICAN COUNCIL ON ADOPTABLE CHILDREN (NACAC)
1346 Connecticut Ave. NW, Suite 229
Washington, DC 20036
(202) 466-7570
(Clearinghouse offering conferences, newsletters, and general information. Subscriber membership: 3800 Market St., Suite 246, Riverside, CA 92501 (714) 788-6423.)

ORPHAN VOYAGE
2141 Road 2300
Cedaredge, CO 81423

POST ADOPTION CENTER FOR EDUCATION AND RESEARCH (PACER)
2255 Ygnacio Valley Rd., Suite L
Walnut Creek, CA 94598
(415) 935-6622
An organization devoted to addressing the lifelong issues of adoption for all triad members.

TRIADOPTION LIBRARY
PO Box 5218
Huntington Beach, CA 92646

Foreign/International Adoptions

AMERICANS FOR INTERNATIONAL AID AND ADOPTION
947 Dowling Rd.
Bloomfield Hills, MI 48013

FAMILIES ADOPTING CHILDREN EVERYWHERE (FACE)
PO Box 102
Bel Air, MD 21014

THE FOREIGN ADOPTION CENTER, INC.
2701 Alcott St., Suite 471
Boulder, CO 80211

FRIENDS FOR ALL CHILDREN
445 S. 68th St.
Boulder, CO 80303

FRIENDS OF CHILDREN OF VIETNAM (FCVN)
600 Gilpin St.
Denver, CO 90218

HOLT ADOPTION PROGRAM, INC.
PO Box 2440
Eugene, OR 97402

LATIN AMERICAN PARENTS ASSOCIATION (LAPA)
PO Box 72
Seaford,NY 11783
(203) 255-6152

DAVID LIVINGSTON MISSIONARY FOUNDATION ADOPTION PROGRAM
PO Box 232
Tulsa, OK 74101

LOS NINOS INTERNATIONAL AID AND ADOPTION REFERRAL
919 W. 28th St.
Minneapolis, MN 55408

LOVE THE CHILDREN
221 West Broad St.
Quakertown, PA 18951

MISSIONARIES OF CHARITY
2562 36th St. NW
Washington, DC 20009

ORGANIZATION FOR A UNITED RESPONSE (OURS)
3307 Highway 100 North, Suite 203
Minneapolis, MN 55422
(612) 535-4829
(Parent support group with bimonthly magazine.)

Child-Free Living

NATIONAL ORGANIZATION FOR NONPARENTS
806 Reisertown Road
Baltimore, MD 21208

ZERO POPULATION GROWTH
1346 Connecticut Ave. NW
Washington, DC 20036
(202) 785-0100

APPENDIX B

U.S. Public Health Service Regional Districts

Public Health Service Region I
John F. Kennedy Federal Building
Boston, MA 02203
(617) 835-1426

Public Health Service, Region II
26 Federal Plaza
New York, NY 10007
(212) 264-2560

Public Health Service, Region III
PO Box 13716
Philadelphia, PA 19101
(215) 596-6637

Public Health Service, Region IV
101 Marietta Tower, Suite 1007
Atlanta, GA 30323
(404) 221-2316

Public Health Service, Region V
300 South Wacker
Chicago, IL 60606
(312) 353-1385

Public Health Service, Region VI
1200 Main Tower Building
Dallas, TX 75202
(214) 655-3879

Public Health Service, Region VII
601 East 12th St.
Kansas City, MO 64106
(816) 374-3291

Public Health Service, Region VIII
19th and Stout Sts.
Denver, CO 80294
(303) 844-4461

Public Health Service, Region IX
50 United Nations Plaza
San Francisco, CA 94102
(415) 556-5810

Public Health Service, Region X
2901 Third Avenue, Mail Stop 501
Seattle, WA 98121
(206) 442-0430

INDEX